A Special Thank You

I would like to thank God for helping me write this book. Every day, I woke up and prayed for Him to give me the words to write.

I would like to thank my family who have been so encouraging during the writing process.

I would like to thank Jalen Barnes for helping me put my thoughts on paper, Ally Hansen for all her hard work in putting this book together, and Peter Korer with Think Ink Printing for doing all of the layout and design.

A Note To My Readers:

There are some things I say more than once in this book, and that's on purpose. It's only after you hear something over and over again that it really clicks. When I repeat myself, it's because I really want to hammer the point home.

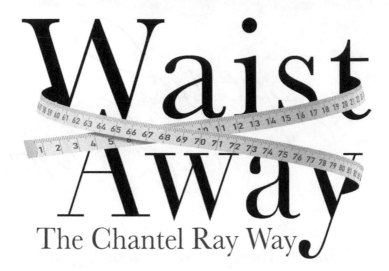

Waist Away

The Chantel Ray Way

Introduction

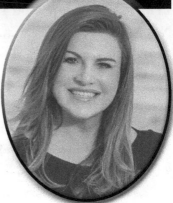

As you pick up this book, you may be asking yourself some questions.

Who is Chantel Ray?

Why should I take advice from her?

Good questions! So, let me tell you a little bit about myself.

My name is Chantel Ray and I run a multi-million-dollar real estate company. I'm not a medical doctor or a nutritionist (red flag!); I actually have my degree in mathematics. I'm a 42-year old mother to a 15-year-old daughter and a six-year-old son. I have a loving husband who owns a competing real estate company and has always called me beautiful even at my highest weight. That leads me to what makes me qualified to write this book you're reading.

I may not be a doctor, nutritionist, fitness trainer or anything like that, but I am someone who, like you, has spent most of her life obsessing over diets and struggling with her weight. If I could gather up all the pounds I've gained, lost, and gained again, I could build a whole new person.

I have tried almost every weight loss strategy that's out there. I've read almost every weight loss book. The topic of weight loss is something I have always been passionate about, even when success escaped me. I'm the kind of person to walk right up to a thin stranger in the gym and ask, "What did you have for breakfast?" You can see how direct I am! What you're reading is the result of my passion to solve the mystery of my own weight loss once and for all.

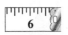

A lot of this book is a combination of information I wrung out of my thin friends, personal research, and the "secret sauce" that finally cracked the code for me and my weight loss. That "secret sauce" is heavily based on the technique known as **intermittent fasting.** You see, I was raised to believe that I could do anything I set my mind to, but for some reason I just couldn't seem to lose weight. This plan that I developed around fasting got rid of all of the complicated dieting rules I struggled with and gave me back control in the one area of my life I didn't have it.

Who am I? I'm the woman who lost so much weight doing diets that people thought I was anorexic, and then I gained it all back. I'm the woman who met 75% of her friends at the gym asking them to text me pictures of what they ate for every meal. I'm the woman who got sick and tired of being in bondage to diets that made me so obsessed with food and counting calories! To be honest, I'm probably you!

If you're sick of trying to find the perfect diet that fits you and you're ready to finally move over and do it God's way, then this is the plan for you! On this plan, you're not going to deprive yourself of the foods that you want. You're going to learn how to listen to your body and regain self-control in your life when it comes to food. When you're finished with this book, you're going to be empowered with the tools to never stress about losing weight again!

Best of luck!
Chantel Ray

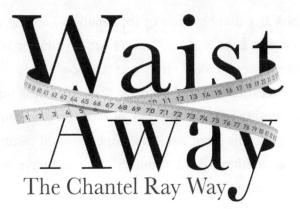

The Chantel Ray Way

One thing you have to understand about the Chantel Ray Way is that it's **not a diet.** That's a good thing! I believe diets are the worst thing ever when you're trying to lose weight. They actually make you *more* obsessed with food. All of the rules and restrictions diets place on you make them too hard to stick to. That's why, no matter how many diets you commit to, you always seem to gain all of the weight back. Here's the thing: any diet works if you can stick to it. However, that's the problem. Diets are NOT sustainable.

Everything you're going to learn in this book is based on the 10 Chantel Ray Way Rules, 10 Biblical Principles, and the practice of intermittent fasting.

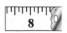

What is Intermittent Fasting?

Intermittent fasting is a pattern of eating where you restrict the number of hours that you eat. In my research, I interviewed over 1,000 thin people and most of them did not have a **specific hour** of the day that they ate (e.g. lunch at 12, dinner at 6). They all ate *naturally* based on when they were actually hungry. Most of them eat one or two meals a day in a window of time we call an **eating window.**

You open your eating window when you consume your very first meal, snack, or caloric drink of the day. You close your eating window after you consume your very last calorie. There is no magic number of hours that every person should use for their eating window. Eight hours works great for some and six hours is better for others. Some eat only one meal and a snack a day in a window of four hours or less. The length of your eating window should be what works best for you with consideration to the portion sizes you eat.

The basis of this lifestyle is this: you don't restrict *what* you eat, but *when* you eat. You can eat whatever you want as long as you only eat in your eating window and follow the 10 Rules and 10 Principles. These Rules and Principles work together with intermittent fasting because if you think you can lose weight by eating non-stop for eight hours straight, then you're sadly mistaken! These Rules and Principles will teach you to **never overeat** and to **eat only when you're truly hungry.**

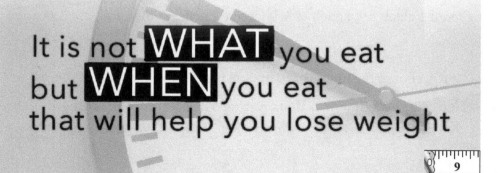

It is not **WHAT** you eat
but **WHEN** you eat
that will help you lose weight

Intermittent fasting requires you to restrict the window of time that you eat rather than track every calorie that you consume. Once you're in your eating window, you can eat what you like so long as you're physically hungry. When the eating window is open, you can eat food and drink caloric beverages. When it's closed, you're fasting and you can only drink water, coffee, and unsweetened tea. Below is a chart with examples of sample eating windows:

Examples of Intermittent Fasting

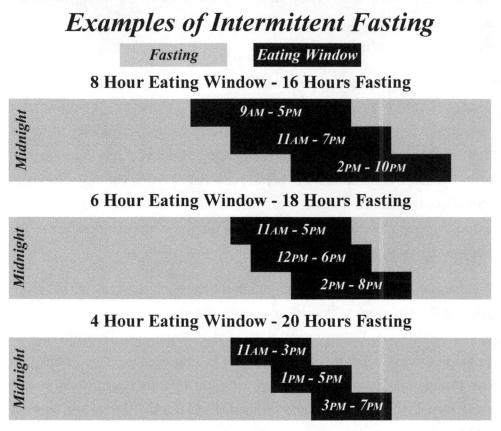

If your eating window is 8 hours long, then that means you're fasting for 16 hours. If you're eating for 6 hours, then you're fasting for 18. This is also called the **clock approach** as seen in the image below.

Clock Approach Example

You choose the times that work best for you! Below are examples.

4 Hour Eating Window **6 Hour Eating Window** **8 Hour Eating Window**

2-6pm, 3-7pm, 4-8pm   *3-9pm,2-8pm, 1-7pm*   *1-9pm,2-10pm, 3-11pm*

When doing the clock approach, I recommend starting off with an 8 hour window, while following the 10 Chantel Ray Way Rules and 10 Biblical Principles. If you don't see yourself losing weight, start reducing your window. As you can see from the chart, if I'm doing the 4 hour fast then I'm only eating from 2-6, 3-7, or 4-8. I'm fasting the rest of the time. With the 6 hour window I'm eating from 3-9 and, again, fasting the rest of the time. The beauty of this approach is that you get to choose the window you want to eat in and what works with your schedule. I have tons of friends that like to eat at night, and some that eat during the day like me. The bottom line is, the fewer hours you eat the more weight you melt away. My eating window is determined by how much weight I want to lose and the sizes of my meals.

The other way you can look at intermittent fasting, besides watching the clock, is what I call the **meal approach**. The meal approach involves skipping one or two meals a day. If you want to melt fat away faster, I have tons of friends that only eat one meal a day. The meal approach is great because you end up picking the meals that you want to eat each day. Here's a sample week of yours truly using the meal approach:

Meal Approach Examples
You Choose The Meals That Optimizes Your Results

	Breakfast	Lunch	Dinner	
Day 1	X	✔	✔	I skipped breakfast because I wasn't hungry and ate a medium-size lunch and dinner.
Day 2	X	✔	X	I went to one of my favorite Italian restaurants called Aldo's. I had a big lunch because I was very hungry from an intense working out earlier that day. That was my only meal for the day.
Day 3	✔	✔	X	Because I had my last meal at 1pm the day before, I was very hungry the following day. I decided to eat breakfast and lunch. I wasn't hungry by the time dinner came around, so I skipped it.
Day 4	X	✔	✔	I skipped breakfast like I normally do and had my usual lunch and dinner as my two meals.
Day 5	X	X	✔	I knew I was going to a late dinner with friends, so I decided to skip breakfast and lunch altogether.

That's a sample meal approach week for me.
Of course, yours might look different.

I typically use the clock approach with my favorite eating window of 12-6pm. I like to eat in that timeframe with a medium-size lunch and dinner, but it doesn't always work out that way. Lately, I've gone a little rogue, and that meal approach sample is what my last couple of weeks looked like.

The number of pounds I lose is directly related to the size of my meals and the hours I eat. The reason that the number of hours you fast and eat have such a dramatic effect on your weight loss, is because of how your body fuels itself. Your body has two options for fuel: glucose (sugar), from the food you recently ate, or fat that's already stored in your body. Your body will always burn sugar first. If there's so much sugar present that your body never needs to burn fat, you won't lose weight because fat-burning is what results in weight loss.

To help you understand what I'm talking about, imagine you have cash in your pocket and cash in the bank. You're not going to drive all the way to the bank to withdraw money if you have some already in your pocket. You're going to use up everything in your pocket first before you ever touch what's in the bank. That's how your body works with sugar (pocket money) and fat (money in the bank). After 18-24 hours of fasting, your body has burned up all of the sugar and starts attacking the fat. That's what you want! This is called transitioning from a sugar-burning mode to a fat-burning mode and I will cover this critical phase in more detail later in the book.

This is what the Chantel Ray Way is all about!

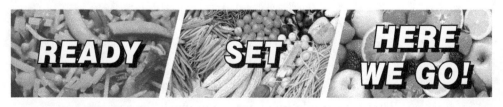

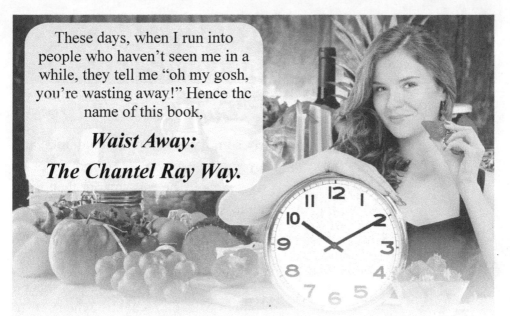

These days, when I run into people who haven't seen me in a while, they tell me "oh my gosh, you're wasting away!" Hence the name of this book,

Waist Away:
The Chantel Ray Way.

Even though my friends noticed the weight loss, I always felt like I hadn't lost much because it was just one or two pounds. Then I realized that a pound of fat is about the size of a can of diced tomatoes. That's actually a lot! I want to encourage you not to dismiss your progress even when it doesn't seem like much. Every pound counts and it's a testament to your hard work. Throw yourself a mini party and reward yourself (not with food). Get a massage, enjoy a hot bath, or do something to congratulate yourself. You deserve it.

Part I - 10 Chantel Ray Way Rules

Rule 1:
Savor the Food

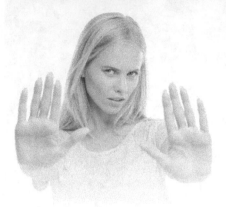

"Stop Eating" Cues

My son, Kyle, is my absolute pride and joy and he eats like a true thin eater. At six years old, he eats smarter than most adults because he doesn't eat anymore than it takes for him to be full. His sense of satiety is very strong. **Satiety** is the feeling of being satisfied.

To help yourself recognize when you're satisfied and not overeat, you need to develop "stop eating" cues. It's like training a dog to go potty. I got a new puppy, Coco, and we had trouble potty training her at first. I discovered bell training and it worked really well. Basically, you ring a bell every time you take her outside to go potty. If you keep doing this, eventually your dog will ring the bell herself when she's ready to go. Ringing the bell is her "go potty" cue.

So, you can develop "stop eating" cues for yourself. Since I have trouble knowing when to stop eating, I have ways to signal my body that it's time to call it quits. Give these a try:

1. **Chew a piece of gum**

2. **Brush your teeth**

3. **Have a cup of tea or coffee**

4. **Flee the scene of the food**

14

Coffee is a good way to end your meal, but you have to be careful because it can have a lot of sugar in it. A coffee from one of the popular coffee shops can have 48g of sugar! I make my coffee with cream and either a little bit of sugar, no sugar, or sugar-free flavorings.

Caution: No Coffee Is Calorie Or Sugar Free Unless It Is Black Coffee!

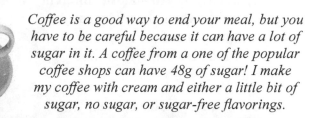

Coffee is a good way to end your meal, but you have to be careful because it can have a lot of sugar in it. A coffee from a one of the popular coffee shops can have 48g of sugar! I make my coffee with cream and either a little bit of sugar, no sugar, or sugar-free flavorings.

Coffee	Size	Milk	Calories	Sugar
Vanilla Latte	16oz	Non-Fat	230	9.5
Hot Chocolate	16oz	Non-Fat	360	10.5
Caffe Mocha	16oz	Non-Fat	330	8.5

Savor Your Food

The best thing you can do to help you decide when to stop eating is to eat what you really want. Savoring your food is easier when you're eating what you really want to eat.

I used to consider taking what I thought was an "easy route" to lose weight - having surgery or doing a fad diet - but I realized that the true solution was to eat real food and never deprive myself. In order to do that, I have to savor my food.

Looking back, I'm shocked at how often I used to eat without even thinking about whether I was actually hungry or not. I ate based on how much food was on my plate. No matter how much food filled the plate, I always ate it all. So, I realized that the problem wasn't with the food itself. Thin eaters eat any kind of food they want and don't deprive themselves.

I also noticed how slowly some thin eaters eat. It can take up to 45 minutes for them to eat their food while it's not hard for me to finish in two minutes! When you eat slower, you taste and **savor** the food.

15

There's a trick to help you eat slower called "One Food at a Time." I want us to try this experiment together:

Go get a plate and put 4 different chips on a plate (EX: Veggie chips, tortilla chips, sour cream and onion chips, nacho cheese chips). Begin to eat the chips and watch what you do. If you take a bite of each chip one after the other, they'll all start to taste the same. If you eat them separately, they'll all taste different and you can decide which ones you really want to eat. Eating one food at a time, lets you savor it and it helps you with portion control.

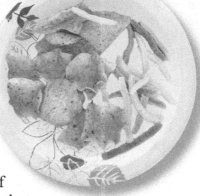

Let's say, for dinner, you have steak, peas, and broccoli. Try eating as much steak as you want and don't touch anything else. Once you eat as much as you want, move on to the peas. After that, eat the broccoli. Instead of switching back and forth, you eat one food at a time. If you do this, you'll only eat what you want and stop when you're full. If you attack everything on the plate, you'll eat more than you need.

I personally LOVE chocolate mousse. Since I particularly like the whipped cream, all I do is take a little whipped cream and a little bit of the mousse and just skim the top of it. I use a fork and just take razor thin slices. I'm savoring it. The goal is to savor your food and not deprive yourself of it. If you're going to eat M&Ms, take one M&M, put it in your mouth and savor it one at a time. Really enjoy the taste. See, you're not depriving yourself! Don't rip the bag open and dump the whole thing in your mouth. Take your time and enjoy it.

Your Fixed Weight Point

If you currently weigh 180lbs but you want to be at 140, then you have to eat the amount of food a 140lb person would eat. The best way to do this is to savor your food. Eat only part of the full plate that you used to eat. As you chew slowly and eat smaller amounts, you're going to change your portion size to match your new fixed weight point.

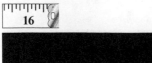

Rule 2:
Never Eat Past 4 on the Hunger Scale

Psalm 63:5 (NLT)
*5 You satisfy me more than the richest feast.
I will praise you with songs of joy.*

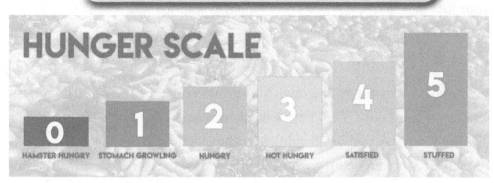

HUNGER SCALE

0	1	2	3	4	5
HAMSTER HUNGRY	STOMACH GROWLING	HUNGRY	NOT HUNGRY	SATISFIED	STUFFED

0 - Hamster Hungry: Starving, ravenous, weak, grouchy. All you can think about is what to eat and how you can get it. You may get a headache, struggle to concentrate, or get "hangry" (hungry + angry).

1 - Stomach is Growling: Empty stomach. You can physically hear your stomach growling and feel an empty sensation. It's important that you feel both sensations because your stomach can growl for other non-hunger reasons like digestion. Be sure that it's growling because it's empty. Everything sounds good to eat at this point of hunger.

2 - Hungry: You're starting to think about food, and certain things sound good to you. You're deciding what your body is craving.

3 - Not Hungry/Not Full: Neutral. You sense that there is some food in your stomach and you're at peace. Your stomach feels comfortable.

4 - *Satisfied/Full:* Comfortably full. You might want to eat more, but you shouldn't.

5 - *Stuffed:* Uncomfortably full. You're getting tired because your body is using all of its energy to digest food. You may want to take a nap or need to unbuckle your belt. You feel as if you've overeaten.

You want to be at a Hunger Level 1 (Stomach is Growling) when you eat your first meal of the day. You don't have to wait for your stomach to growl to eat your second meal, but you do need to make sure that you are at least at a level 2 (Hungry).

Learning to wait for your stomach to growl is one of the most important aspects of this entire plan! I even debated naming this book, *True Hunger* or *Thin Eater!* A thin eater only eats when she's truly hungry. If you put food in front of her, no matter how amazing it is, she won't eat it if she's not hungry. My friend, Christy, is a perfect definition of a thin eater. I've tested her several times with some amazing food.

"Try this! Taste this!" I said while putting food in front of her. She responded the same way every time. She told me she wasn't hungry and could save it for later.

The term hamster hungry (Level 0) came from a friend of mine who owned a pet hamster that had three babies. One day, she went out of town and forgot to feed the hamster. She came back to discover to her horror that the mama hamster had eaten her babies! That's *hungry!* I allow myself to get a Level 0 when I'm on a Biblical fast, but I have to control myself and not overeat. You can never overeat, even when you're hamster hungry. In the section on fasting (Principle 3), you'll learn how to cry out to God and ask Him to remove the urge to run to food and overeat.

How to Be A Skilled Thin Eater –
Stopping Before You're Full

1   ***Don't Eat Until You Feel Tired.*** You should still have energy when you're done eating. If you're dozing off on the couch after dinner, you ate too much.

2   ***Get the Food Out of Sight.*** When you're full, stop eating and get the food away from you. If you're at a restaurant, ask for a to-go box. If you're at home, put the leftovers in your fridge. Pray for God to remove the desire to eat anymore food.

3   ***Change Your Definition of Full.*** Fullness shouldn't feel uncomfortable and your stomach shouldn't be extended.

4   ***Understand the 20 Minute Principle.*** Understand that it takes 20 minutes after eating to realize that you're actually full. Always stop before you're satisfied so your body signals can catch up.

5   ***Remember the Consequences.*** You know all of the negative consequences overeating brings. You know how uncomfortable it makes you feel. You don't want to go back to that ever again.

5 Steps for Slowing Down When You Eat

1 **Pray.** Before you eat, quote Psalm 81:10.

> ### Psalm 81:10 (NIV)
> [10] I am the LORD your God, who brought you up out of Egypt. Open wide your mouth and I will fill it.

Then say, "Lord, you know that I want to eat really fast so I ask you to help me slow down. Help me chew every bite. I ask you to fill my heart and mind so that I'm not ravenous. Help me to feel calm, slow down, put my fork down after every bite. In Jesus' name, "amen."

2 **Take a Break.** Pause in the middle of your meal to do something else. Go to the bathroom or get a refill on your drink. Ask if anyone needs something from the kitchen. Find a way to step away from your food. My friends teased me all the time for not taking a breath when I ate. Don't be like that!

3 **Use a fork and knife.** Eat your meals with utensils so you can cut up your food into small bites.

4 **Dissect your food.** My thin friends start to pick apart their food and eat only what they enjoy when they approach that "satisfied" feeling. Take one of my favorites, a chocolate mousse, for example. I like the whipped cream and I don't care for the crust on the bottom. So, I'll barely skim the edge of the meringue with the whipped cream and chocolate. I dip my fork so it's barely full and put it in my mouth. I skim for the best parts. Do the same thing. Use slow, "up and down" repetitive motions and take your time to enjoy it.

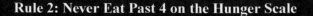

20

5   ***Savor Every Flavor.*** If you eat a piece of dessert or decadent chocolate, take a single square or piece of it and savor it. Don't chew and swallow it right away. Let it sit there. Notice the different textures and how it melts in your mouth. Let it linger as long as you can. Even when you're drinking coffee, take a sip of it and savor it.

Thin eaters know how to eat just beneath what their bodies are calling for. That's how they stay the same weight day in and day out. I have an aunt who's been wearing the same clothes for 35 years because of this! Don't eat a single bite more than what you need. The difference in you being thin and overweight can be determined by just a few calories a day.

Using the calorie calculator at calculator.net, you can see the difference a few calories a day can make. A 40 year old person at 5'4" eating 1940 calories a day weighs 130lbs. The same person eating 1877 calories a day weighs 120lbs. That's a difference of only 63 calories!

How Many Calories Should I Eat To Maintain My Weight If I'm A 40 Year Old Woman?

Weight	Calories
130	1,711
135	1,743
140	1,774
145	1,805
150	1,836
155	1,867
160	1,899
165	1,930
170	1,961
175	1,992
180	2,023
185	2,054
190	2,086
195	2,117
200	2,148

How Thin Eaters Eat

After 20 years of research on how to lose weight, I decided to follow thin eaters around for 24-48 hours and observe everything they ate and how they ate it.

I went out to lunch with one woman to Burger King. She got a Whopper with cheese and fries and so did I. I ate my Whopper, my fries, and a whole milkshake before she even finished half of her burger. I was completely finished, still feeling hungry, and hoping I could find a way to eat the rest of her food!

I asked her why she didn't eat the whole burger. She said, "I don't want anymore. I'm done." When I asked her if she felt guilty for wasting the food, she said she could waste it in the trash or waste it on her hips. She wasn't greedy for more food than what her body was asking for and because she ate what she wanted all the time she wasn't desperate for the burger. On the other hand, I restricted myself to grilled chicken and salads all the time and went crazy for the burger because I didn't know when I was going to have one again.

Another time, I went to a salad bar with a thin friend. My office is right across from Whole Foods, so my friend came to visit me and we walked over. She added beets, pumpkin seeds, and broccoli and so did I. I copied the amounts exactly. She didn't even know what I was doing; she assumed we just liked the same foods! We sat down to eat and my salad was gone in 4 minutes. I looked up and she had only eaten half of hers because she was busy talking. She took the rest home to eat later. While she ate, she practiced all of the principles. She prayed before she ate, paused to talk, and dissected her food. I saw her pick up pumpkin seeds and pop them in her mouth.

Watching thin eaters eat is very powerful. It's something you should try. However, don't get the wrong idea when you see a thin eater eat a big meal. Thin eaters will change how much they eat day to day based on what their body calls for. Some days they eat more than others but they never overeat.

Rule 3:
Don't Eat Your First Meal of the Day Until Your Stomach Growls

> ## 1 Corinthians 9:27 (NLT)
> *27 I discipline my body like an athlete, training it to do what it should.*

Wait for the Growl

> ## Psalm 81:10 (NIV)
> *10 I am the Lord your God, who brought you up out of Egypt. Open wide your mouth and I will fill it.*

The best time to eat is when your stomach is **growling**. That's when your stomach is actually hungry. It's like a fuel gauge on a car. Your body will let you know when it's time to eat the same way a car does when it's on "E." The drop in blood sugar that occurs when you're truly hungry sends a message to your stomach to produce that empty "growling" sensation.

That's the biggest thing I learned about thin eaters. They never eat before that stomach growl unlike emotional eaters who eat for any reason at all. When you want to eat before you're truly hungry, that's the time to quote your scriptures. You have to learn to eat when you're *physiologically* hungry (your body is hungry) and not when you're *psychologically* hungry (your brain is hungry).

I congratulate myself when I successfully wait for true hunger to eat.

23

"Great job, Chantel, you waited until you were physically hungry to eat!" Reward yourself with positive self-talk when you make the right decisions.

This eating plan is all about *when* you eat rather than *what* you eat. Your stomach growl is your signal to start your eating window. You'll train your body to an eating schedule as you continue to do this. If you don't get a growl when you're supposed to, then you know you ate too much at your last meal. It's possible to go 48 hours without a stomach growl when you overeat, because you ate too much on your last binge. If you're overweight and a chronic overeater, you might not have a real sense of hunger because you're running on fat and your last meal. Keep the amount of food that you're eating small so that you're hungry the next time you eat. Don't delay your eating window indefinitely if you don't hear a growl. I don't recommend you go longer than 36 hours without eating something small.

I found that there's a stigma with people about letting their stomachs growl. Stomach growling is a good thing! Getting hungry is okay! We act like being hungry is the worst thing in the world when it isn't. It's your body's natural signal to eat. Let your body get hungry, and then feed it. If you don't hear your stomach growl at least once a day then, Houston, we have a problem! I can't stress this enough. Your first meal of the day doesn't begin until your stomach growls.

God designed your body to teach you when it needs food. The sad thing is there are people who have never heard their stomachs growl because they never let themselves get hungry. Every chance they get, they're shoving food in their mouths.

You can start your eating window only after your stomach growls, but you still shouldn't eat immediately. This is because you're in fat burning mode when your stomach growls. That's your time of maximum weight loss potential and you want to prolong that for a little while. When your stomach first starts to growl, I suggest you have a cup of black coffee or unsweetened iced tea to get you at least an hour past that growl.

Coffee: The Appetite Suppressant

Coffee is a great way to get you through your fast. Coffee and unsweetened tea act as appetite suppressants. We have to discuss coffee for a minute because the biggest problem people have with this is that they don't want to drink black coffee under any circumstances!

"I *have* to drink coffee with cream in the morning," they tell me. "That is just a must! If I can't have coffee with cream in the morning, this diet is not for me."

You should not consume any calories while you're fasting and that includes coffee with cream. That being said, I have plenty of people on this diet who are doing coffee with cream in the morning. Believe it or not, you can still get results. I have an aunt who is 5'4' and 98lbs, and eats exactly this way. She drinks coffee with cream multiple times a day until about 1pm. However, she only ever has 1-1½ meals after that. She eats very, very little.

I don't recommend coffee with cream because I believe it will slow down your progress and keep you from discovering true hunger. I prefer you dig in and learn to take it black or try unsweetened tea instead. Eighty percent of the fat loss battle is controlling your hunger and coffee is a great way to stave off hunger until you're ready to eat.

There is a timing to when you should drink coffee as well. Don't drink it as soon as you wake up. You're not usually starving when you first get out of bed. Save it for later on when you feel hunger setting in but you need to push on with your fast a little longer. That's when coffee and tea are a great help.

I recommend no more than 2-3 cups of coffee a day. If you drink more than that, the coffee won't be as effective in suppressing your appetite.

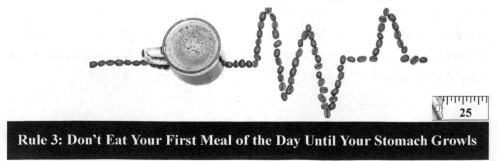

Rule 3: Don't Eat Your First Meal of the Day Until Your Stomach Growls

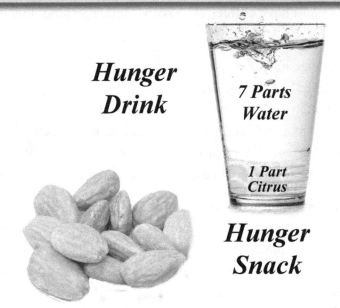

Hunger Drink

7 Parts Water

1 Part Citrus

Hunger Snack

I have a "training wheels" trick you can use if you're new to fasting. It's not something you want to use forever. Otherwise, it will become a crutch. If you find yourself getting hungry before it's time to start your eating window, or if you want to push past your stomach growl a bit, make a **Hunger Drink.** It's very easy to make: mix 7 parts water and 1 part orange, lime, or lemon juice. Sips of this will help you power through.

Hunger snacks can only be consumed inside your eating window. They're meant to be high-protein, high-fat snacks that keep you from being ravenous. The best hunger snacks you can pick are nuts like cashews or almonds. If you can't find something high in fat, then look for a high-fiber food. Good options are an apple with peanut butter, half of an avocado, a pickle, or an egg. Don't make your hunger snack a processed, high-carb food.

Rule 3: Don't Eat Your First Meal of the Day Until Your Stomach Growls

Rule 4:
Pick An Eating Window And Stay In It

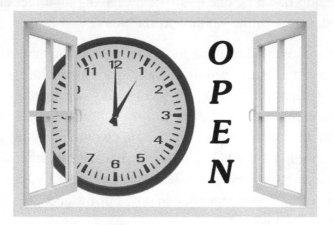

An eating window is a specific period of time in which all of your caloric food and beverages must be consumed. Your eating window opens as soon as you take your first bite/sip of food of the day. The eating window closes after you've taken your last bite/sip of food for the day. If that's six hours after your first meal, then that was a six-hour eating window.

Let's say it's Monday and you have a six-hour eating window scheduled. You decide to eat your first meal at 1pm. That clock starts after you take your first bite of food at 1. Everything you eat after that has to happen before 7pm. After that, you're done eating until you start your next window tomorrow. Now, suppose you finished eating dinner by 7pm, but you decide to have a glass of wine or a bowl of ice cream at 9pm. Well, you just extended your window into an eight-hour window. You can't mark that day as a successful six-hour eating window. No calories can be consumed outside of your eating window. Everything counts.

I first heard about intermittent fasting from my trainer, Chris Sykes. He lost 20lbs in two weeks and we had a mutual friend that lost 30lbs in 60 days. Chris explained to me that I could eat whatever I wanted. All I had

27

to do was confine myself to an eight-hour eating window. I thought that it didn't sound too hard at all. That was because I was already used to eating nine hours a day even though I didn't know it at the time. After two weeks of trying the eight-hour window, I didn't lose any weight. I realized that cutting my eating down by one hour wasn't having an effect on me. So, I decided to reduce my eating window to six hours.

Pay attention to how you respond to the eating window and how you can transition over time. Some people are going to start with the eight-hour window, realize that it's too easy for them, and jump to six hours. Others will start with eight, move to seven, and then down to six. I moved from eight to six quickly when I realized eight hours wouldn't cut the mustard for me to lose weight like I needed to. Now, my normal eating window is from 12pm-6pm. I listen to my body and learn the days that I'm hungry and the days that I'm not. It'll vary from day to day. For instance, the week before my period I'm a lot hungrier.

What you want to avoid is eating more than your body needs. No matter how long your eating window is, you can't overeat. If you eat from 12-6 (a six-hour window), but you consume a huge lunch, a snack in the middle, and a huge dinner then you're still eating too much. I learned quickly that if you overeat, you still won't lose weight no matter how short your window is.

You'll find out what works for you and that will change over time. I think the window that works best for most people is a 5-6-hour window with one medium-sized meal and one small meal.

The wonderful thing about fasting is that your body learns to expect food at a certain time of day. Around 11 or 12 o'clock, my stomach growls because it's used to eating around that time. Because of this I'm not constantly thinking about food and that's one of the major goals of The Chantel Ray Way. Once my eating window is closed, it's closed! At that point, I have mentally shut myself down from thinking about food and it's so peaceful! If you've never experienced this before it may sound unbelievable, but trust me when I say it's a much better way to live.

I feel much more productive now that I'm not constantly thinking about food. I get so much more done and I don't even want to start eating because once I do, I know I'm going to slow down. I'm not tired when I fast. There's a myth that you get tired if you don't eat, but the opposite happens. I have more energy when I don't eat than when I have frequent meals all day. I think it's because the body takes so much energy to digest food. When I fast it's not doing that all day.

Believe me, there are going to be days when you get tired of this plan and think, *"this is too much!"* The first couple of months on this plan have a lot of moments like that. Find the eating window that works for you and remember that you don't have to restrict anything in your diet. This isn't a plan that deprives you.

Get rid of the concept of the "cheat day." Remember that you aren't depriving yourself. Once in a blue moon, usually when I have a special event like a wedding to attend, I'll have an eight-hour eating window and eat less throughout the day. You may have days like that too, but you're not going to be doing cheat days.

There's definitely an adjustment period, but it's something you can do. I had a lot of friends that thought they could never do this, but once they saw me lose weight they changed their tune.

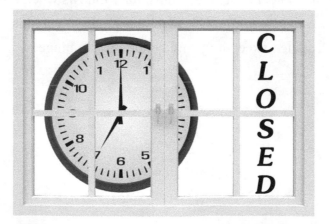

Rule 4: Pick An Eating Window And Stay In It

The Flexibility of the Eating Window

Different people like to do different things when it comes to the timeframe of the eating window. Some prefer to start eating in the morning and others in the afternoon. I prefer to fast in the mornings and so I get push-back from people who insist on telling me that skipping breakfast is *soooooo* bad for me. I haven't seen any negative consequences yet.

When you do find the timeframe for your eating window, stick with it. The people I know who are the most successful with this plan pick a designated time of day for their eating window that they keep consistent. If you do it the same time every day, your body gets used to it and it makes it easier.

If you ever get off track, you may need to make adjustments. One day, I had an early lunch at 11:30am. Since I chose to eat, I ended up eating in a seven-hour window instead of the six-hour window I was scheduled to have. I balanced myself back out by swapping in an additional four-hour eating window day in place of one of my six-hour windows. This also helps me on days when I overeat. My body benefits from the "cleanse" of a shorter window.

As an additional note, I do a lot of four-hour windows when I really want to jumpstart my weight loss after I've hit a plateau. If you do this, don't overdo it or you'll struggle to keep it up and be tempted to binge.

Eating Window Alternatives

An eating window isn't the only way to employ the principles we discuss in this book and get results. You can simply wait until every stomach growl to eat, but I think it becomes difficult to plan your life around the growls when unexpected events and outings with friends come up. However, that method will most certainly result in weight loss just like eating windows will.

I interviewed over a thousand thin people for this book and I learned that while not all of them participated in intermittent fasting, their eating behavior contained one or more of the following attributes:

- **Eating one meal a day (sometimes two)**

- **Eating in a six hour window**

- **Eating in an eight hour window, very clean**

- **Eating only when the stomach growls**

- **Eating 100 calories or less in the morning**

Every single person I interviewed did at least one of these things. They all got themselves to a fasted state at some point in the day. Whether they know it or not, there's an element of intermittent fasting in the way they eat.

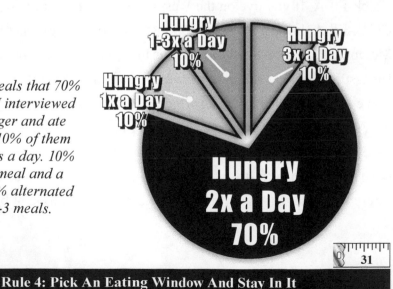

This graph reveals that 70% of the people I interviewed felt true hunger and ate twice a day. 10% of them ate three times a day. 10% ate one big meal and a snack and 10% alternated between 1-3 meals.

Hungry 1-3x a Day 10%

Hungry 3x a Day 10%

Hungry 1x a Day 10%

Hungry 2x a Day 70%

31

One of my favorite places to go is the The Ritz-Carlton in Key Biscayne, Miami. The last time I visited, I interviewed thin ladies, as usual, to find out what they were eating for every meal. It was surprising to learn that a higher-than-normal percentage of women were eating three times a day. I dug deeper and realized that they were eating clean for 95% of their diet or higher; they also ate very small portions. One other thing they told me is that they ate a high-protein snack 20 minutes before a meal to keep them stable. These snacks included raw nuts like cashews and almonds (usually 10 at a time) or peanuts (usually 20). It kept them from getting hamster hungry and helped them control their eating.

Save Your Food

Proverbs 25:28 (NIV)
28 Like a city whose walls are broken through is a person who lacks self-control.

I was talking to one of my friends about this plan and she said it would never work for her because her favorite thing in the world is breakfast at Chick-Fil-A. If you live on the West Coast you may not be so familiar with Chick-Fil-A, but it's a really good fast food restaurant where I live. Unlike McDonald's, Chick-Fil-A only serves breakfast food during morning hours. I reassured her that she didn't have to give up Chick-Fil-A breakfast food. She could schedule her eating window to start in the morning when Chick-Fil-A was serving breakfast or she could pick up the food in the morning and save it for when she's ready to start her window. There are times when I've been craving breakfast food all day, so I cook it for dinner for my family. There's no rule that says you can only eat breakfast food at breakfast time!

Today, I scheduled myself to eat from 12:30-6:30pm because I have people coming over for dinner at 5:45. For lunch at my office we had catering from a place I had been dying to try called Zoe's Kitchen. The food arrived around 11am, so I went and took exactly what I wanted to eat – beef skewers. I made my plate and let it sit on the edge of my desk until 12:30 when I was ready to eat. Then I heated it up and ate it.

My naturally skinny friend, Christy, does that. We have something called Thursday Fundays when everybody brings food. Christy loves my guacamole (I make the best guacamole in town). After a couple of Thursday Fundays, I noticed that Christy would take a big scoop of guacamole and stick it in the refrigerator. I was confused about what she was doing. Was she hiding the guacamole? I finally asked her what was going on and she told me that she was putting the guacamole away until she was hungry. It was a good plan because whenever I bring guacamole in, it goes in 20 minutes!

The same thing happened with my lunch today. I took the beef skewers and made my plate early. I wanted to make sure I could have them later. Just to see what would have happened if I waited to fix my plate, I went to check out the buffet again around the start of my eating window. Sure enough, only kernels of food were left.

You have to believe that you can control yourself around food. Recently, I had a breakfast meeting from 10am-12pm. At 10, everyone ordered and ate. I waited until 11:30 to order and ate after everyone else. Even when I got my food, I wasn't hungry. I set it aside for about 20 minutes and ate it later. It's really empowering when you do stuff like that!

Rule 4: Pick An Eating Window And Stay In It

Social Scenarios

Let me give you a scenario: you have a breakfast date with friends in the morning and then a dinner for work at night. You're committed to a six-hour window, so there's no way you can eat at both. What do you do? These social scenarios pop up all the time and you have to make a decision. When am I going to eat and when am I going to say no?

I went out to breakfast with some friends the other day and I knew I had a dinner to go to that same night. I chose not to eat at breakfast. I wasn't even hungry, but my friends kept pushing me to eat and telling me to "get something small" because "we hate to eat without you."

I put my foot down and refused to eat because, #1) I wasn't hungry and #2) I could sit there without being worried about the "pull" of food. I was at breakfast to enjoy my friends' company. I could even talk more with them because I wasn't stuffing my face with food. Remember, you can always order food and save it for later.

Let's talk about "not worth it" moments. Let's say you ate from 12-6pm on a Friday, and later that night one of your girlfriends invites you out for dinner and drinks. That is a "not worth it" moment! If you can't handle the temptation then it's better not to go. If you can, then go and enjoy yourself without food. Have a soda water or something without any calories. Something I like to do is have a glass of soda water with five lemons and five limes squeezed and the lemons and limes taken out afterward.

Rule 5: *Eat the Best First*

Psalm 81:16 (NLT)
[16] *But I would feed you with the finest wheat.*
I would satisfy you with wild honey from the rock.

Thin eaters only eat what they really, really love. I interviewed tons of thin eaters and they told me that they actually **taste** and **rate** each food on their plates. The average eater tastes something she doesn't like and eats it anyway because she feels she has to "clean her plate."

Imagine a plate of steak, mashed potatoes, broccoli, and a salad. The average eater eats the foods she likes least first and saves the best for last. The thin eater eats whatever she likes the best *first* because she knows that she's going to stop eating once she gets full. If she likes the steak and mashed potatoes, she's going to eat that instead of feeling forced to eat the broccoli and salad she doesn't want. She eats what she craves.

Usually, a salad is served before the main course of any meal. Sometimes we eat it not because we enjoy it, but because it's there. When the main course comes out – and, be honest, that's the food you showed up for – you eat more of that to satisfy your craving and end up eating past full. Afterward, you blame it on the meat and carbs in the main course when it's actually the salad that's the problem. You could have refused to eat that entirely and waited on what you actually wanted and eaten less overall.

Start rating not just the foods on your plate, but even the parts of each food. I like edges of brownies instead of the middle. So, I should just eat the edges only. I don't have to eat the whole thing, just the best part. This is why thin eaters always leave some food on their plates. They are not part of the "clean your plate" club.

Some people say you're required to eat everything on your plate because there are starving children in other parts of the world. I don't believe that. All of the extra food we eat is causing heart disease, diabetes, and more.

Is it better to get health problems because you're overeating or to just throw the food away?

35

Exodus 16:1-5 (NIV)

¹ The whole Israelite community set out from Elim and came to the Desert of Sin, which is between Elim and Sinai, on the fifteenth day of the second month after they had come out of Egypt. ² In the desert the whole community grumbled against Moses and Aaron. ³ The Israelites said to them, "If only we had died by the Lord's hand in Egypt! There we sat around pots of meat and ate all the food we wanted, but you have brought us out into this desert to starve this entire assembly to death." ⁴ Then the Lord said to Moses, "I will rain down bread from heaven for you. The people are to go out each day and gather enough for that day. In this way I will test them and see whether they will follow my instructions. ⁵ On the sixth day they are to prepare what they bring in, and that is to be twice as much as they gather on the other days.

What's key in that passage is that God said to only eat what fills you up for that day. You don't need to be greedy and continue to eat more. That doesn't mean that you can't have leftovers. It means you're only eating enough to fill your body.

To make sure that you're only eating what you really want, use the:

Chantel Ray Way Enjoyment Scale:

★ Not very good at all.

★★ Ehh. It's not bad, but it's not good.

★★★ Pretty good. Just OK tasting.

} *Not Worth Eating*

★★★★ Party in my mouth. It's REALLY REALLY good.

★★★★★ *BEST THING I'VE EVER HAD.* My absolute favorite bite.

On a scale of 1-5, you want to only eat foods that are a 4-5 level of enjoyment. You shouldn't even waste calories on anything beneath that. If the steak and potatoes are your 5s, eat them first. Once you're full, you don't have to eat anything more. You're done!

My friend, Christy, went on vacation to Italy. When she got back I asked her if she gained or lost weight. She ate pasta every night and she lost four pounds! How is that possible? Well, she never ate breakfast and they walked everywhere they went. She ate pasta every night for seven nights, but she never overate. Christy likes pasta, but on average she only eats it 1-2 times a week when she craves it. She doesn't eat anything that's not a 4 or 5 on the enjoyment scale.

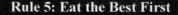

Rule 6: Eat What You Really Want

No Restrictions

Dietary restrictions kept Jewish Christians from initially accepting Gentile Christians into their fellowship. Peter's vision in Acts 10:9-16 presented the new rules of eating.

Acts 10:9-16 (NIV)

⁹ About noon the following day as they were on their journey and approaching the city, Peter went up on the roof to pray. ¹⁰ He became hungry and wanted something to eat, and while the meal was being prepared, he fell into a trance. ¹¹ He saw heaven opened and something like a large sheet being let down to earth by its four corners. ¹² It contained all kinds of four-footed animals, as well as reptiles and birds.¹³ Then a voice told him,

"Get up, Peter. Kill and eat."
¹⁴ "Surely not, Lord!" Peter replied.
"I have never eaten anything impure or unclean."
¹⁵ The voice spoke to him a second time,
"Do not call anything impure that God has made clean."
¹⁶ This happened three times, and immediately the sheet was taken back to heaven.

38

This removed the dietary restrictions that God placed on Israel through the Mosaic Law as seen in Leviticus 11:

Leviticus 11: 1-8 (NIV)
[1] *The LORD said to Moses and Aaron,* [2] *"Say to the Israelites: 'Of all the animals that live on land, these are the ones you may eat:* [3] *You may eat any animal that has a divided hoof and that chews the cud.*
[4] *"'There are some that only chew the cud or only have a divided hoof, but you must not eat them. The camel, though it chews the cud, does not have a divided hoof; it is ceremonially unclean for you.* [5] *The hyrax, though it chews the cud, does not have a divided hoof; it is unclean for you.* [6] *The rabbit, though it chews the cud, does not have a divided hoof; it is unclean for you.* [7] *And the pig, though it has a divided hoof, does not chew the cud; it is unclean for you.* [8] *You must not eat their meat or touch their carcasses; they are unclean for you.*

It goes on even longer than this in Leviticus and in Deuteronomy 14. Under the New Covenant, the restrictions were lifted and we were instructed not to try to force anyone else to eat a certain way.

Romans 14:2-3 (NIV)
[2] *One person's faith allows them to eat anything, but another, whose faith is weak, eats only vegetables.* [3] *The one who eats everything must not treat with contempt the one who does not, and the one who does not eat everything must not judge the one who does, for God has accepted them.*

We have to respect each other enough to let each other eat the way we think we should.

> ## Romans 14:14 (NIV)
> *14 I am convinced, being fully persuaded in the Lord Jesus, that nothing is unclean in itself. But if anyone regards something as unclean, then for that person it is unclean.*

If you want to be vegan, be vegan. If you want to be vegetarian, be vegetarian. Do you want to be paleo? Be paleo. You have to decide for yourself. I am not going to judge people who eat differently from me, and they shouldn't judge me. Our focus should be to take care of our bodies because they are God's temple.

> ## 1 Corinthians 3:16 (NIV)
> *16 Don't you know that you yourselves are God's temple and that God's Spirit dwells in your midst?*

We can serve God effectively when we're healthy. Chasing after fad diets is like chasing the wind. We need to control our appetites and let the Holy Spirit direct our decisions.

> ## Ephesians 5:18 (NIV)
> *18 Do not get drunk on wine, which leads to debauchery. Instead, be filled with the Spirit.*

> ## Mark 7:15 (NIV)
> *15 Nothing outside a person can defile them by going into them. Rather, it is what comes out of a person that defiles them.*

Too Clean

Don't try to overdo it by eating 100% clean all the time. A lot of dieters have blacklisted certain foods with the belief that, if you eat them, you won't lose weight. In my experience, trying to eat super-clean prevented me from losing weight. What happened was that I ate perfectly Monday through Friday, but when the weekend came along, I completely lost it. Instead, I suggest writing in a food diary the things you eat. People who track their food in a journal lose more weight than those who don't. It's not something you have to do forever, but it's a good idea to start out with.

The problem with making your food "behave" is that if you restrict all foods but protein in order to lose weight, then that's what you'll have to do for the rest of your life. That's unreasonable! Instead, you want to change your habits to how true thin people eat. It's making yourself behave instead of your food. You can still eat the foods you love while losing weight, and nothing is unacceptable to eat. The things you want to avoid are sugars and chemicals. Keep those in the realm of the three bite rule.

It's all about self-control. Even if you're eating healthy, you can still overeat and consume too many calories. When I was trying to eat really clean, I found these healthy chips that I loved to eat. They were dairy-free, gluten-free and every other type of free. They were only 160 calories a serving. The problem was that I would eat the entire bag in one sitting. That was five servings! Just like that, I had consumed 800 calories. I could have just had 200 calories of Doritos and been better off!

One thing I want every reader to understand, is that as long as you eat in your eating window, you can't make a mistake no matter what you eat. Yesterday, I had a half of a donut and didn't feel guilty about it one bit. The problem with dieting is, people don't want to control how much they eat, so they make their food behave. They overeat on things like carrots or celery and say that because it's healthy food it "doesn't count." That's not what the Bible says at all. The Bible says to put a "knife to your throat" if you're being gluttonous. Period. The End. You have to practice self-control.

41

Rule 7: *How Big is the Differential?*

> ## 2 Timothy 1:7 (NIV)
> [7] *For the Spirit God gave us does not make us timid, but gives us power, love and self-discipline.*

Caloric Intake

Maybe you heard the story that came out a few years ago about John Cisna, the science teacher who ate only McDonald's for six months and lost 56lbs. He did this on a 2000 calorie diet while walking 45 minutes a day[1]. Moral of the story? Caloric intake is a BIG deal!

You need to start eating what you want and not what you think you should eat. Imagine you're at lunch with your girlfriend. You choose the full-size Caesar salad and she chooses the lunch special cheese pizza. Who just ate the most calories? You did! The cheese pizza from the average restaurant is 950 calories while a Caesar salad can be as much as 1280 calories. Crazy, right? You can get so caught up on trying to eat healthy and think you're doing good when really you're missing out on eating what you really want for no reason.

My trainer told me that people trip themselves up in a similar way when it comes to exercise. You can work out at the gym and overestimate how many calories you actually burned – treadmill calorie counters are not accurate! So, say that you *think* you burned 400 calories in a workout when, in reality, you only burned 200. If you go out and devour 400 calories based on that misperception, you're suddenly in a bad place. I'm not an advocate for counting calories. I *am* an advocate of getting yourself to a place where you eat less food. That's the whole idea. We've fed our bodies too much and too often. Now, we're limiting the amount of times that we're eating and the amount of food that we're eating with this plan.

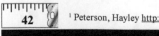

42

[1] Peterson, Hayley http://www.businessinsider.com/how-to-lose-weight-eating-only-mcdonalds-2015-10

Caloric intake is very important. My aunt weighed 125lbs for the longest time before she dropped to 90lbs and stayed there. Using the calorie calculator at calculator.net, I can estimate that she only had to go from eating about 1800 calories a day to about 1524 to maintain that weight loss. It's unbelievable! Just a small change in your caloric intake can make such a difference.

It's not very hard to reduce calories and still eat what you love. You can do it easily with sandwiches. In my opinion, there's never really a time you should be eating two pieces of bread. One is more than enough. If you can get away with it, have an open-faced sandwich with just one slice of bread. To reduce the bread on an English muffin, scoop out the middle part. It tastes better that way, in my opinion, because I like the crunchy part anyway. You can do a similar thing with a bagel and take out the entire middle part. This way, you get rid of a lot of calories but still feel like you have a nice sandwich.

On the other hand, there are times when you're craving something and you need to let yourself feel satisfied. In Virginia, there's a restaurant called Baker's Crust that has something called the "Gotta Have It" burger and sometimes I GOTTA HAVE IT! That kind of burger isn't quite as good without the bun, so, when I eat it, I eat the whole thing. You don't want to make every meal a mental battle. It's really exhausting. People that are naturally thin don't do that to themselves; counting calories, asking *can I?* or *should I?*…all of that is just mentally exhausting.

Are All Calories Created Equal?

When you do this intermittent fasting plan correctly, you're going to consume less calories and that equals weight loss. If you're worried that eating the decadent foods you want is going to counteract that, check out this story.

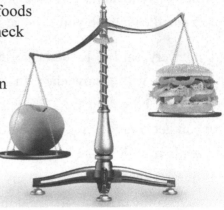

Mark Haub is a professor of human nutrition at Kansas State University who, for a class project, ate junk food for the majority of his diet and lost 27 pounds in two months[2]. The key? He restricted his calories to less than 1800 a day. It didn't matter that he was eating mostly Twinkies, Doritos, Oreos and more. The calorie deficit led to his weight loss.

Now, if you had one person eat 1800 calories of Twinkies vs 1800 calories of grilled chicken, I do think you would see a difference in muscle definition. However, if your focus is weight loss, proper intermittent fasting helps you get where you want to be. Also, because intermittent fasting involves eating windows, and, as a result, less meals a day, it removes the need for being overly focused on counting the actual calories. If you eat one meal a day, for example, it's very difficult to eat more than 1200 calories in one sitting.

Macronutrients

Macros (short for macronutrients) are nutrients your body needs to survive. They are fats, proteins, and carbs. All three of these are needed for cognitive function, energy, and more. Protein really ties into lean muscle mass and satiety (the feeling of being satisfied). If you're deficient of protein, it can contribute to weakness, mood changes, lack of concentration, and joint issues. By simply listening to your body, evaluate if you're getting enough of everything you need. Don't get obsessive with trying to count every last gram.

[2] Park, Madison. http://www.cnn.com/2010/HEALTH/11/08/twinkie.diet.professor/index.html

Know Yourself

Let's say I really wanted some chocolate mousse, but, in an effort to be healthy, I tell myself, "I'm just going to have this apple with almond butter instead because that's the healthier option." Sometimes, that will work, but often times it really depends on how badly you want it. Because what you don't want to do is eat that apple with almond butter, say, "that just didn't do it!" and go eat the mousse anyway. Now, you've eaten the apple, almond butter, and the mousse! You've eaten all those calories! It's better to just eat the mousse in a small amount rather than overeating.

In my opinion, no one ever needs an entire donut. It's way too much sugar. But does everyone need a couple of bites of donut every once in awhile? Absolutely. In the beginning, it takes time because you have to tell yourself that you can eat just 3 bites and be done. When you're starting out you're probably going to have to throw away half of the donut to keep yourself in check.

Scales

Two days ago, I got on the scale and I gained two pounds. Today, I got on the scale and lost 3lbs. Did I really lose 3lbs? No. That's why the scale isn't a good indicator. **Don't freak out over the scale.** It will drive you up the wall, mentally. It could be something as simple as water that makes your scale weight fluctuate. I recommend weighing once a week, and **only when you're feeling thin**. If you're feeling bloated, then don't get on the scale. I only get on the scale if I think I've lost weight. Otherwise, why am I going to get on the scale just to feel bad about myself? No way.

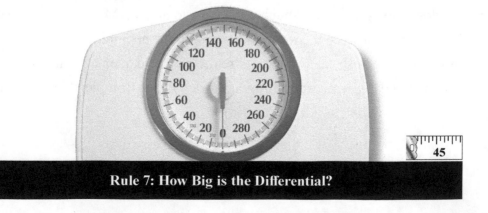

45

Rule 8:
Remember the Law of Diminishing Returns

Proverbs 27:7 (NIV)
⁷ One who is full loathes honey from the comb, but to the hungry even what is bitter tastes sweet.

Everything tastes amazing when you're really hungry! Notice that when you take the first bite, the food tastes really great. The second bite is kind of good and the third bite isn't very good at all. Every bite after the first goes down in quality. If you were to rate taste on a scale of 1-10, the first bite is a 10, second bites are a 9, third bites an 8 and on and on. When it gets to a 7, you should be ready to stop eating. Absolutely at 6, you shouldn't be eating it anymore.

Thin eaters eat only what they love. Everyone else eats the entire plate no matter what. We don't even pay attention to whether it still tastes good or not.

Thin eaters say, "This doesn't taste that good anymore. I've had enough."

Picture a donut and see how you can divide it into 8 pieces. The maximum you should be eating is 3-4 bites. You got the taste, you got the flavor, you're good now! You don't need to eat the whole thing. Literally, throw the rest of the donut away. In the beginning, you have to do that. Maybe later on in this journey you can keep the rest for later, but in the beginning you just need to throw it in the trash can. And if you're the kind of person to go into the trash can later and dig it out, then throw it farther away! Completely get rid of it!

Rule 9: *Portion it Out*

My 96-year old grandmother recently offered me some of her antique china. I looked at the size of the dishes and was shocked by how small the plates were. The average plate we eat from in our homes today is twice the size of those dishes my grandmother used. Nowadays, we are eating portions that are way too big. Since our stomachs are the size of a fist we want to be eating meals that are no bigger than that. Now, if you're eating one meal for the day, your portions will be bigger but they should always be reasonable.

Plates *used* to be this size...

Now they are this size!

Portion Control

A tip to control your eating portions is to cut your food into halves or quarters. When you eat a burger, cut it into pieces like a pie. Eat two or three pieces instead of the whole thing.

47

Tracking Calories

"Chantel, I'm fasting and eating in my window and doing everything just right, but I'm STILL not losing weight! What's wrong?"

If you're not losing weight, then you're eating too many calories. You can fast and eat in a six-hour window all you want, but if you're still consuming a massive amount of calories, you won't lose weight. The whole idea is to get a total daily calorie deficiency.

Today, I did the You Pick Two® from Panera Bread. I got half of a chicken panini and a cup of broccoli and cheddar soup (600 calories) and I ate some of the bread that comes with it (200 calories), plus two Chia bars™ (100 calories each), which puts me at 1000 calories so far today. That was a very big meal - bigger than I usually eat - so now I only want to have 400-500 calories for the rest of the day. In fact, because I'm so satisfied now, I might not eat at all for the rest of the day.

Now, I roughly calculated those calories in my head and I don't recommend counting calories as a practice. This is only something you want to do if you're not seeing results. But let's not get consumed with calories unless we're not seeing results. It's at that point that you need to be honest with yourself and admit that you're eating more than you should be.

> **1 Corinthians 6:12b (NIV)**
> *[12] "I have the right to do anything"—*
> *but I will not be mastered by anything.*

It's important that you decide what a reasonable amount of food to eat is beforehand and decide to put the rest away. Restaurants typically give you way too much food. Your stomach is the size of a fist. Most restaurants give you four or five "fists." Get yourself down to two fists and take the best parts of whatever you're eating. Remind yourself that you're going to get hungry again and don't think you have to just eat, eat, eat!

Don't have the attitude that *I only have six hours to eat! I have to eat as much as I possibly can because I'm not going to be able to eat again until tomorrow.* Approach your food like a thin eater. It's about balance. If you used to eat a big pasta dish for lunch, balance it out by adding vegetables or protein. I try to have protein with every meal. Almost half of everything I eat is one-half protein. It keeps me satiated.

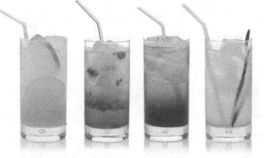

Drinking Calories

I noticed that I don't lose weight when I drink my calories. I have to even be careful with green juice because there are calories in that too. The rare times that I drink alcohol I drink it with zero calorie mixers like diet tonic and soda water. With wine, I only suggest low sugar organic wines without a ton of preservatives. Keep in mind that all of this still has to happen in your eating window. Just because the calories are in a drink doesn't mean they don't count!

Rule 10: *Use the 3 Bite Rule*

> ### Proverbs 25:16 (NLT)
> *16 Do you like honey?*
> *Don't eat too much, or it will make you sick!*

When you cut out entire food groups and limit the amount of calories you consume, you have to rely on your willpower to succeed. At some point your willpower kind of gives up! Anytime I go the route of completely banning a particular food from my diet, I go crazy and I start losing my willpower. One day, I just explode and eat everything in sight! But when I have one or two bites of decadent foods I can say, "OK, I had it, it was fine, the end." It makes me feel like I can still have what I want.

I've discovered that the magic number for me to have the decadent foods I want is three bites, two times a day. Eating three bites of dessert doesn't make my body respond negatively.

This is something I can do and maintain my weight. If I'm aiming to lose weight, then I might do this once a day or even not at all. However, I never ban myself from eating any particular food. That behavior always leads to a binge somewhere down the road. Allowing myself three small bites satisfies the craving.

Once again, if you don't have physical ailments, you can eat whatever your body craves. I have tons of skinny friends who eat whatever they want all the time, but because they fast, they still maintain and lose weight. I have one particular friend that weighs 100lbs and drinks 1-2 sodas a day! She's an intermittent faster and she only eats one meal a day! This proves that the amount of food you eat is the most important factor in your weight loss. You can overeat on any diet and still be overweight.

50

Part II
The 10
Biblical
Principles

Principle 1: *Never Overeat*

Proverbs 23:2 (NIV)
*and put a knife to your throat if
you are given to gluttony.*

Ezekiel 16:49 (NLT)
*Sodom's sins were pride, gluttony, and laziness,
while the poor and needy suffered outside her door.*

Proverbs 23:20-21 (NASB)
*Do not be with heavy drinkers of wine, Or
with gluttonous eaters of meat; For the heavy
drinker and the glutton will come to poverty,
And drowsiness will clothe one with rags.*

Do you want to know the #1 reason losing weight is so complicated for all of us? It's because we're eating too much dang food! We literally eat every hour and that includes snacking. If you look back at our ancestors, they didn't do that. Food wasn't as easily accessible-for them as it is for us in 21st century America. Back then, food had to be found, taken, prepared, and then eaten. They weren't eating four to five small meals a day like some diets out there suggest. They didn't have refrigerators to store that much food. I honestly believe that our bodies are hardwired to be able to go without food for a much longer time than we allow ourselves to. Overeating is what's made us sick and fat. Overeating is such a major issue that the Bible mentions it quite often. In Scripture, it's called **gluttony**.

Gluttony and Laziness

Words like "gluttony" and "laziness" aren't very popular in the Christian world. The reason we shy away from these topics is because so many Christians are lazy and gluttonous.

Deuteronomy 21:18-21 (NASB)

If any man has a stubborn and rebellious son who will not obey his father or his mother, and when they chastise him, he will not even listen to them, then his father and mother shall seize him, and bring him out to the elders of his city at the gateway of his hometown. They shall say to the elders of his city, 'This son of ours is stubborn and rebellious, he will not obey us, he is a glutton and a drunkard.' Then all the men of his city shall stone him to death; so you shall remove the evil from your midst, and all Israel will hear of it and fear.

Ouch! Sounds harsh right? In the Old Testament, you could stone someone for being this rebellious! Obviously, we don't live under Old Testament laws anymore thanks to Jesus, but I like that this passage points out how serious we should be taking these issues. This is important to God, but we don't take it seriously in the Church today and we have overweight leaders who won't touch the subject. We all just laugh it off like it's not a big deal. That has to stop. Gluttony is **sin** and it's something we MUST talk about!

Acts 26:18 (NASB)

to open their eyes so that they may turn from darkness to light and from the dominion of Satan to God, that they may receive forgiveness of sins and an inheritance among those who have been sanctified by faith in Me.

Principle 1: Never Overeat

10 Ways to Avoid Overeating

1. ***Order an appetizer.*** When you're eating out, ordering a small appetizer to share is a good idea. Have your appetizer 15-20 minutes before your meal arrives. Once you start eating your meal, you can eat with a lot more control because you'll already be approaching that full feeling.

2. ***Talk, talk, talk***. Try putting your fork down and have a conversation with the people you're eating with. It's easy to overeat when you eat so fast that you're basically inhaling your food.

3. ***Ask God to help you slow down***. Ask for help before you start eating. I believe God has a great sense of humor because any time I say that prayer, something always happens to slow me down. One time, my son asked me for carrots, so I had to get up from the table to get them. Once I got back, I could only take one bite before my husband asked for ketchup. After I got the ketchup, the doorbell rang! It was funny, but the Lord answered my prayer.

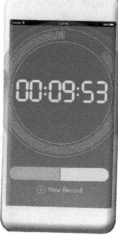

4. ***Set a timer.*** Set a timer for two minutes, take a couple of bites, and then stop. Look up from the food and give it time to hit your bloodstream. Take the time to talk or take a bathroom break. This will give your brain time to register that it's full before you clean your whole plate.

5. ***Use a knife and fork.*** Think of all the food you ate today. Did you use a knife and fork at any point? We eat a lot with our hands which can contribute to overeating. Start using a knife and fork with your meals to control your portions. If you're eating a pizza, cut it up into tiny pieces. You can do this with just about any food.

6. ***Sip hot tea.*** Sip hot tea in between bites of your meal. It breaks your eating rhythm and slows you down.

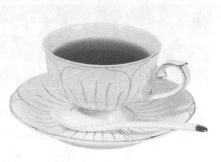

7. ***Take smaller bites in general.*** I'm someone who likes to do everything big, so I used to take big bites, too. Now, I find that it's actually fun to take a sandwich and cut it up into tiny pieces and eat it that way.

8. ***Get the food out of sight.*** The second you start feeling a little bit full, you need to get rid of the food in front of you. Call the waitress and get a to-go box right away. If you're at home, move your plate to the kitchen and start boxing it up immediately. The longer you sit there with the food, the more you're going to be tempted to take another bite and another bite and another bite even though you're not hungry.

9. ***Dissect the food.*** Let's pretend you're eating sushi. Visually dissect the sushi and pick what you consider to be the best parts. Is it the little sesame seeds? Is it just the meat? Pick it apart and eat the parts you actually want and enjoy. Nibble and savor each little pinch until you're full. Don't eat all the things you don't want just because you feel like you have to.

10. ***Use a Smaller Plate.*** Filling up a small plate tricks your brain into thinking you're getting a lot more food than you are. At the same time, you're downsizing your portions. Your brain thinks you're piling it on, but you're eating less because it's a smaller plate.

Principle 2:
Recognize True Hunger

Psalm 63:5 (NLT)
*⁵ You satisfy me more than the richest feast.
I will praise you with songs of joy.*

Hunger and Fullness

You have to get in tune with your body and ask, "How hungry am I? How full am I?" This is the only way you're going to successfully lose weight with intermittent fasting. When you learn how to evaluate **true hunger**, you're going to discover you don't need to eat as much food or as many meals as you think you do. You might end up only eating one or two meals a day.

Now, don't look at that and think, "That's crazy! I might as well give up now." You're going to find out what works for you, and as you learn your true hunger you're going to find yourself eating less and less. Start with learning not to eat more than what your body needs. To help you do that, I developed the **Hunger Scale**. The next time you think about eating food, locate your level of hunger on this scale first.

The Hunger Scale

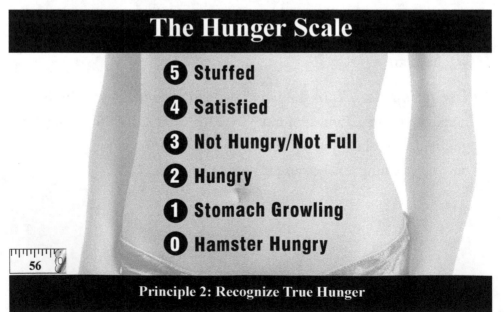

- **5** Stuffed
- **4** Satisfied
- **3** Not Hungry/Not Full
- **2** Hungry
- **1** Stomach Growling
- **0** Hamster Hungry

56

Hunger Scale Definitions:

0. ***Hamster Hungry:*** Starving, ravenous, weak, grouchy. All you can think about is what to eat and how you can get it. You may get a headache, struggle to concentrate, or get "hangry" (hungry + angry).

1. ***Stomach is Growling:*** Empty stomach. You can physically hear your stomach growling and feel an empty sensation. It's important that you feel both sensations because your stomach can growl for other non-hunger reasons like digestion. Be sure that it's growling because it's empty. Everything sounds good to eat at this point of hunger.

2. ***Hungry:*** You're starting to think about food and certain things sound good to you. You're deciding what your body is craving.

3. ***Not Hungry/Not Full:*** Neutral. You sense that there is some food in your stomach and you're at peace. Your stomach feels comfortable.

4. ***Satisfied/Full:*** Comfortably full. You might want to eat more, but you shouldn't.

5. ***Stuffed:*** Uncomfortably full. You're getting tired because your body is using all of its energy to digest food. You may want to take a nap or need to unbuckle your belt. You feel as if you've overeaten.

You NEVER want to get to this level!

Let Your Stomach Growl

I only eat when my stomach is growling because that's when I know my body is actually hungry. It's like a fuel gauge on a car. You fill up your car when it hits "E" and you eat when your stomach growls. I've learned that thin people wait for the stomach growl because they associate that with true hunger. Emotional eaters eat because they're tired, bored, stressed, or whatever! You want to eat when you're *physiologically* hungry not when you're *psychologically* hungry. In other words, eat when your body is hungry, not just when your brain is hungry.

There's a difference between the growl of your stomach digesting your food and the growl of your stomach being empty. When you feel that second growl, be excited!

"Great job, Chantel, you waited until you were physically hungry to eat!" I say things like this to myself to encourage good eating habits. Every time you wait until your stomach growls to eat you should reward yourself with positive self-talk.

(Insert your name here), you did a great job!"

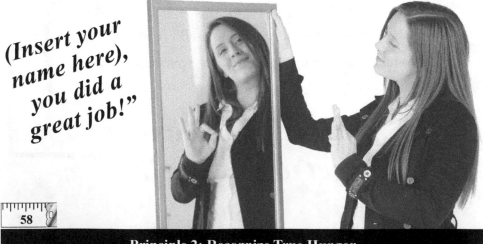

58

You're capable of bypassing your initial hunger pangs and waiting until true hunger to eat. In fact, wait until a couple hours after the growl, if you can. The longer you wait to eat, the further you're pressing into that fat burning zone. You'll eventually train your body to get used to an eating schedule - mine is 12-6pm. Obviously, I don't always keep that schedule because if I go to a nice dinner, then it's usually going to be after 6pm. On those days, I might extend my window to an eight-hour window, or I might start my window at 2pm with a light snack and be done by 8 or 9.

If you're not hearing a growl, then that more than likely means you ate too much at your last meal. It's possible to go as long as 48 hours before reaching "stomach hunger" when you come off of a binge. Most people never hear their stomach's growl simply because they're constantly eating; they never actually reach an empty stomach. Keeping this in mind, you should make smaller meals so that you can reach that point of true hunger. If you eat the right amount of food, you will be hungry when it's time to eat again. It's important to create a habit of getting hungry. All of that being said, if you reach 36 hours without hearing a growl, you should go ahead and eat something small.

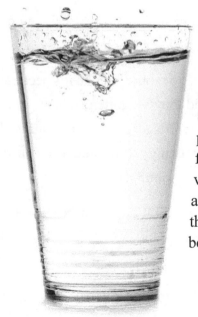

There's one small thing you should avoid when you're eating: don't drink too much water. Drinking too much water while you're eating your meal can actually dilute your stomach acid and interfere with your digestion. You want everything working properly so you can sense hunger and fullness. However, outside of your eating window, you can drink as much or as little as you want. Let your body tell you when it's thirsty just like when it's hungry. When your body is hungry, eat. When it's thirsty, drink.

Rocket science, right?

Defining Hunger

The crux of this entire book is the proper understanding of hunger. To understand hunger, you have to properly define it. **Hunger is the physical need for fuel.** It's something that comes in cycles. You're never hungry all the time. Hunger is also something that we often confuse with appetite. **Appetite is your mental desire for food.** You can have an appetite all the time. If you come back to work after your lunch break and someone brings in donuts, you might eat one. That's not hunger; that's appetite. Most people never know their true hunger because they don't let themselves get hungry. The goal with intermittent fasting is to let yourself get hungry. We want to be excited about getting hungry!

When you're truly hungry, you know exactly what your body is craving and what you want to eat. On the flip side, when you're not hungry, a friend can ask you what you're in the mood for and you have to decide. That opens the door to unnecessary eating.

When you eat according to true hunger, you're not eating when the clock tells you to. There is no more, "it's 12 o'clock, that's lunch time!"

It takes about a week to figure out true hunger. For some people, it's because they've never heard their stomachs growl and they've gotten so heavy that they could probably go without eating for days. Hunger can also be confused with dehydration. You can think you're really hungry when actually you're thirsty. Staying hydrated will help you learn your hunger.

You should only ever eat at a level 3 or below. You don't eat because the clock says it's lunchtime and everyone else is going out to eat. You wait until your stomach growls and your body is physically hungry for food.

Here's a perfect example of a thin eater. One of my favorite desserts is

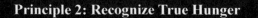

coffee crumb cake. One of my friends knows that I love this, so she made a homemade cake just for me and brought it to the office. The way that I used to be, I would have eaten that cake just so I wouldn't hurt her feelings.

The new me doesn't do that. "That is so sweet of you to make a coffee crumb cake for me," New Me says, "but I'm not physically hungry right now. So, I'm going to save this for later. I'm sure I will love it and I'll text you as soon as I eat it to tell you how much I do." She might press me to try it, but I'm going to stand firm.

Defining Fullness

I never really understood what the definition of full was before I began this journey. I always felt like I was hungry and could eat all day. Sometimes, I would come home from work and, if I was wearing a tight dress, I would change into pajamas so I could eat more at dinner. I don't do that anymore! Now, full is a "polite feeling" for me. Instead of eating until I'm full, I eat until I'm "barely full" or "satisfied." Stuffed and satisfied feel different. If you're eating to the point that you have to take off your belt or change into your pajamas, then that means you're eating *beyond* full.

I learned my biggest lesson on fullness from one of my thin friends - my hairdresser, Danielle. One day in conversation, I discovered that she only eats one slice of pizza for lunch every day. I asked her if that really filled her up and she told me it didn't. She explained to me that when she finishes that slice, even though she's not full, she will be 20 minutes later.

Thin people don't eat to get full. I've learned that they actually hate being full. They don't like the way it feels. You have to adjust your definition of full and not expect the kind of "full feeling" you're used to. Don't be the kind of person who eats faster so she can taste more food before she's too stuffed to eat anymore. There's a real science to understanding when you're truly full and truly hungry, but it's something you'll learn intuitively.

Thin Eaters and Fullness

I mentioned my thin hairdresser who taught me about fullness. In all of my research, I learned that "thin eaters" have certain eating characteristics that revolve around how they perceive fullness. Thin eaters wrap up their food when they're done eating and do it without arguing, pouting or complaining. They know that they'll get hungry again eventually and they don't want to feel stuffed.

It's also important to learn to eat slower so you can sense when your body is full. If you eat too fast, you'll blow right by "just enough" before you realize it.

There's a balance to figuring out when you're full. On days that you're only eating one meal a day, you're tempted to get really, really full to compensate but you can't do that. Even if you're someone who works out and has more muscle mass, you can't use the fact that you need more calories as an excuse to binge. It's important that you create a habit of getting hungry. If you're feeling especially hungry when you sit down to eat, take time to calm yourself so you're not going wild on your food. Use a timer and measure how long it takes you to eat your food.

62

Principle 3: *Fast On A Regular Basis*

Matthew 6:16 (NIV)

[16] *"When you fast, do not look somber as the hypocrites do..."*

All over the Bible there are mentions of fasting. In fact, fasting is mentioned in Scripture, in some form, over 70 times. Notice how in Matthew 6:16 (above) that Jesus says *"when* you fast" (emphasis mine). Apparently, God never intended for fasting to be optional in our lives. It's something He actually expects us to do, and God never tells you to do something you can't do.

I believe there are some walls in life that we won't break through without fasting. Fasting is a Believer's secret weapon. What you have to understand is that this weight loss battle isn't a natural fight. It's a spiritual one. Spiritual battles require spiritual weapons and fasting is one of the most powerful tools in your arsenal. So, don't count it out!

Ephesians 6:12 (NIV)

For our struggle is not against flesh and blood, but against the rulers, against the authorities, against the powers of this dark world and against the spiritual forces of evil in the heavenly realms.

A good analogy about the power of fasting is scuba diving. When you're just looking at the surface of the water from the outside, you can't really see what's going on underneath the surface. It's only after you dive underneath that everything changes. You can see the coral and all the different colors and kinds of fish. It's like everything comes alive! Fasting does that for your spirit. The body is hungry, but the spirit is sharp and everything comes into focus. It makes it easier to hear from God. Fasting definitely needs to be a part of our Christian practice.

63

> ## Matthew 6:16-18 (NIV)
> *"When you fast, do not look somber as the hypocrites do, for they disfigure their faces to show others they are fasting. Truly I tell you, they have received their reward in full. But when you fast, put oil on your head and wash your face, so that it will not be obvious to others that you are fasting, but only to your Father, who is unseen; and your Father, who sees what is done in secret, will reward you.*

The purpose of fasting is not so that you appear spiritual, it's so that you *are* spiritual. It's something you don't have to tell everyone about except for your spiritual partner. You don't need to make a big deal out of it and have a "poor me" attitude. Sometimes, you might just have to tell people, "I'm not eating right now." In the beginning, fasting is NOT a pleasant experience simply due to the fact that you're denying yourself. However, the results are so incredible that once you get past some of the discomforts, you'll see that breakthroughs can happen. Every major breakthrough I've gotten in my life has been a result of fasting. I don't ever get into a serious project or make any major decisions without prayer and fasting first.

It's important to know that fasting doesn't move God. It moves *you* closer to God. It makes things clearer. When you eliminate food, your spirit becomes uncluttered and more tuned in like an antenna. It's like turning the dial and getting a real clear frequency.

When we fast, we're literally denying our bodies of food for a spiritual purpose. It's not dieting. You also have to take that time where you would

64

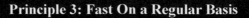

normally be eating and commit it to a spiritual activity. Pray, meditate the Word of God, or worship. While you're fasting, your body is going to throw a fit and tell you that it's hungry, but this is a time when you're denying your physical needs so your spiritual needs can be met.

Fasting also makes a lot of extra time available to you that you used to spend preoccupied with food. While you're fasting, you're not thinking about food, going to the store to get food, or preparing food. Maximize that spare time by spending it with the Lord and see how big of a difference it makes. Take advantage of this time to lean on Him for the strength you need to make it through the fast. Around the same time most days, my assistant, Ally, and I will start to feel really hungry like we want to break our fasts early and eat. So, we stop what we're doing and pray together, asking God for the power we need to push through.

Something that's really important in someone's spiritual growth is the habit of solitude with God. As an early riser, I find my best time to be alone with God is in the morning. I can go to the gym and then have 30-45 minutes alone with God. I ask him for strength to help me not overeat and meet my goals for the day. Your time of day may be different, but it's important to have that. There are so many different things you can do during that alone time with God. You can read a Christian book or listen to Christian music, but the absolute best thing you can do is have total solitude with God and His Word. You want to listen to what He's saying. The back of this book has every Bible verse that we mention in these pages. You can just take that and read them over and over.

65

Colossians 3:16a (NLT)

16 Let the message about Christ, in all its richness, fill your lives....

This scripture is one you need to memorize. This is the key to what should be happening while you're fasting. You're not just saying "no" to food. You're saying "yes" to God. You're choosing Him and His Word to fulfill you instead of food and snacks. Here's a prayer you can pray while you're fasting:

> *"God, you say in your word in Colossians 3:16 that I should be filled with Your words and that is what I'm asking right now; fill me up with Your words from my head to my toes."*

You can quote God's Word for any situation in life. Again, use the resources in the back of this book for ammunition. Whatever verse is appropriate for you in the situation you're dealing with is what you need to feast on and carry with you.

It may seem a little tacky, but you can write verses on your hands with a marker to keep them in front of you. It's actually a great testimony because people will ask what it is. I'm going to write Colossians 3:16 on my hand right now. Today, I'm going to a Mexican restaurant for lunch and I know that one of my weaknesses is the chips. I'm going to ask God to give me the strength to not overeat and choose instead to be filled with His Word.

Lastly, there's one thing you should know about making the decision to fast: some people are going to give you kickback. They'll tell you all about how you're ruining your metabolism by not eating or how it's bad that you're missing breakfast because it's the most important meal of the day. You'll definitely encounter opposition, but remember what I said about dipping beneath the surface. God can speak to you in a still, small voice and you see things clearer when you're not eating. I believe that God speaks to you more clearly when you're fasting. That's not to say He doesn't speak to you when you're not, but it's like gaining clarity. It increases the intensity and focus of your prayers. There is POWER in fasting.

Reasons to Fast:

To Prepare for Ministry

Matthew 4:1-2 (NIV)
⁴ Then Jesus was led by the Spirit into the wilderness to be tempted by the devil. ² After fasting forty days and forty nights, he was hungry.

When Jesus fasted for 40 days, He was getting prepared for His work. Fasting is something you can do to prepare for God's next mission for you.

To Seek Wisdom

Acts 14:23 (NIV)
²³ Paul and Barnabas appointed elders for them in each church and, with prayer and fasting, committed them to the Lord, in whom they had put their trust.

Like Paul and Barnabas, you can use prayer and fasting to seek wisdom for important decisions.

To Grieve

Nehemiah 1:3-4 (NIV)
³ They said to me, "Those who survived the exile and are back in the province are in great trouble and disgrace. The wall of Jerusalem is broken down, and its gates have been burned with fire."

Fasting is even a way to help deal with your grief.

To Seek Deliverance

Ezra 8:21, 23 (NIV)

21 There, by the Ahava Canal, I proclaimed a fast, so that we might humble ourselves before our God and ask him for a safe journey for us and our children, with all our possessions. 23 So we fasted and petitioned our God about this, and he answered our prayer.

Ezra declared a corporate fast for all of the people as they believed God for protection from their enemies on their 900 mile trek.

To Repent

Jonah 3:4-5,10 (NIV)

4 Jonah began by going a day's journey into the city, proclaiming, "Forty more days and Nineveh will be overthrown." 5 The Ninevites believed God. A fast was proclaimed, and all of them, from the greatest to the least, put on sackcloth. 10 When God saw what they did and how they turned from their evil ways, he relented and did not bring on them the destruction he had threatened.

To Worship God

Luke 2:37 (NIV)

37 and then was a widow until she was eighty-four. She never left the temple but worshiped night and day, fasting and praying.

She fasted as an expression of her love for God.

To Gain Victory

> ## Judges 20:26-30,35 (NIV)
>
> [26] *Then all the Israelites, the whole army, went up to Bethel, and there they sat weeping before the LORD. They fasted that day until evening and presented burnt offerings and fellowship offerings to the LORD.* [27] *And the Israelites inquired of the LORD. (In those days the ark of the covenant of God was there,* [28] *with Phinehas son of Eleazar, the son of Aaron, ministering before it.) They asked, "Shall we go up again to fight against the Benjamites, our fellow Israelites, or not?"*
>
> *The LORD responded, "Go, for tomorrow I will give them into your hands."*
>
> [29] *Then Israel set an ambush around Gibeah.* [30] *They went up against the Benjamites on the third day and took up positions against Gibeah as they had done before.*
>
> [35] *The LORD defeated Benjamin before Israel, and on that day the Israelites struck down 25,100 Benjamites, all armed with swords.*

This is what you're doing. You're gaining victory over eating. You're crying out to God for victory in this area and you're going to win!

What Fasting Does

People fast from many different things, but when it's mentioned in the Bible it's all about food. Some of the most important reasons we should fast are for healing, protection, and wisdom.

> ## Isaiah 58:4 (NIV)
> *⁴ Your fasting ends in quarreling and strife, and in striking each other with wicked fists. You cannot fast as you do today and expect your voice to be heard on high.*

In this passage of Scripture, God is rebuking the people for fasting incorrectly. However, if we pay attention, we see the important purpose for fasting: to have our voices heard by God. By fasting, we come into God's presence in a really powerful way. Much of my life is "go go go!" and "do do do!" Fasting is the opposite, though. I'm really focused on the Lord during that time and it bonds me a little bit closer to Him. I feel like I'm really in His face and He's listening.

> ## Isaiah 58:5a (NIV)
> *⁵ Is this the kind of fast I have chosen, only a day for people to humble themselves?*

Again, we see another detail about fasting. It's an activity that humbles you. It sharpens your mind and you can see clearly in a way you couldn't before. Remember the scuba diving analogy? You can't see much above the surface, but, once you dive underneath, a whole world of detail is open to you.

I tell people all the time that fasting is like running. It's something you work at and progress with over time. If you're not a runner, running a block will leave you winded. However, if every day you increase your distance, block

70

by block and mile by mile, you will get stronger. Once you're up to two miles, running a block is easy. Give yourself that time with fasting and let your body gear up to it.

A typical Biblical fast is probably over a 24 hour period. In that time, you reach out to God and say, "Lord, I can't do this on my own. I've tried every diet and every method to break free of this eating struggle. I realize I have put food over you. I'm putting my inability and failure at your feet. I need you to get involved and help me because this is a massive area of struggle for me."

That's humbling yourself before God. We try to live the Christian life in our own power when we don't humble ourselves. Fasting breaks the chain of addictions and problems that we can't seem to break on our own.

In 2 Corinthians 12:1-10, Paul talks about a physical issue he suffered and the conversation he had with God about it.

> **2 Corinthians 12:8-9a (NIV)**
> [8] *Three times I pleaded with the Lord to take it away from me.* [9] *But he said to me, "My grace is sufficient for you, for my power is made perfect in weakness."*

Like many of us, Paul pleaded for God to take the problem away. We all have something in our lives - a struggle or health issue - that we can't beat without God's help. He is the One who can save us.

> **3 John 2 (NIV)**
> [2] *Dear friend, I pray that you may enjoy good health and that all may go well with you, even as your soul is getting along well.*

There are times when we're sick, but God is still the Great Physician and Healer today.

71

> **Exodus 15:26 (NIV)**
>
> *26 He said, "If you listen carefully to the Lord your God and do what is right in his eyes, if you pay attention to his commands and keep all his decrees, I will not bring on you any of the diseases I brought on the Egyptians, for I am the Lord, who heals you."*

God is your healer! 1 Samuel 1 tells the story of a woman named Hannah who fasted in grief because she was unable to bear children. She prayed and asked for God to remedy the problem and remove the stigma of not being able to get pregnant.

> **1 Samuel 1:19-20 (NIV)**
>
> *19 Early the next morning they arose and worshiped before the Lord and then went back to their home at Ramah. Elkanah made love to his wife Hannah, and the Lord remembered her. 20 So in the course of time Hannah became pregnant and gave birth to a son. She named him Samuel, saying, "Because I asked the Lord for him."*

God listened to her prayers through fasting and gave her what she asked for.

The Intermittent Fasting Plan

The Chantel Ray Way is based on the practice of intermittent fasting (IF). There are many diets that use IF with varying rules of what you can and can't eat. The Chantel Ray Way will be different from others you may have heard about. To understand what intermittent fasting is and how we're going to do it, you should know about all of the different kinds of fasting.

The Five Kinds of Fasts

- *Normal Fast* - On a normal fast you are going without food for a defined period of time. You can still have liquids, but without sugar: water, unsweetened tea, coffee (black), etc.

- *Juice Fast* - A juice fast is liquids only but without sugar or calorie restrictions. You're drinking mostly green juice but not having any solid foods whatsoever.

- *Absolute Fast* - When you're on an absolute fast, you are having no food or water at all. I don't think anyone should do this kind of fast for more than 3 days outside of an instruction from God where He promises to supernaturally sustain you.

- *Partial Fast* - Partial fasts specifically omit certain foods. A good example of this is a Daniel fast where you can eat fruits and vegetables among other things but meats are prohibited.

- *Rational Fast* - On a rational fast, you omit certain families of foods of nutrients for designated periods of time. For example, you might only eat protein every fourth day.

Theoretically, you could do any one of these fasts intermittently, but The Chantel Ray Way is strictly a **normal fast.** We'll be alternating between eating windows and fasts. While you're fasting, all food is off limits. That includes drinks with sugar and artificial sweeteners. The best way to put it is to say that while you are fasting you should not be consuming any calories at all.

73

True Fasting

Fasting is the greek word *nésteia* meaning "not to eat." I take that literally, so I'm not a fan of people abusing partial fasts like the Daniel Fast. I see people refraining from meat but overeating on everything else. If you're still eating burritos with cheese and refried beans and salads with more dressing than salad, I don't call that fasting. If you're scarfing down huge portions of bean burgers and bread, I think you're missing the point. The point of fasting is to not eat. When you fast, you make a sacrifice to God first by giving up food for a period of time.

When Daniel chose not to eat meat and wine for ten days, it was because the food was being offered to idols and eating it would have been a sin. So, he ate vegetables and water.

Daniel 1:12 (NIV)
12 *"Please test your servants for ten days: Give us nothing but vegetables to eat and water to drink.*

If someone restricts themselves to just vegetables for ten days, I do see that as a sacrifice. But there's a difference between doing that and finding other ways to overeat and indulge your flesh with everything that falls into the "not-meat" category. A lot of Christians do a version of the Daniel Fast that they say is based on the second time Daniel fasted in Daniel 10:2-3.

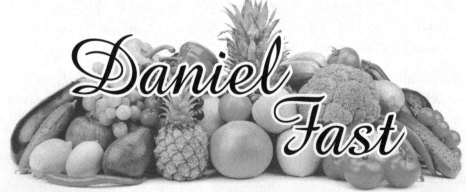

> ### Daniel 10:2-3 (NIV)
> *² At that time I, Daniel, mourned for three weeks. ³ I ate no choice food; no meat or wine touched my lips; and I used no lotions at all until the three weeks were over.*

So, people avoid meat and wine, but overindulge in other things like bread. I'm sorry, but bread is a **choice food**! I've seen people eat processed bread with more chemicals in it than the meat they're avoiding.

The purpose of fasting is to deny your flesh's desires. In order to really hear God, your flesh has to be silenced. By fasting, you tell your flesh who is boss. You tell your body that you're taking charge with the help of Christ. I believe that true power only comes when you fast 100%. Take all the time you spend preparing, eating, and thinking about food and focus it on God: that's when you get results!

> ### Galatians 5:17 (NIV)
> *¹⁷ For the flesh desires what is contrary to the Spirit, and the Spirit what is contrary to the flesh. They are in conflict with each other, so that you are not to do whatever you want.*

Talking About Your Fast

> ### Matthew 6:17-18 (NIV)
> *¹⁷ But when you fast, put oil on your head and wash your face, ¹⁸ so that it will not be obvious to others that you are fasting, but only to your Father, who is unseen; and your Father, who sees what is done in secret, will reward you.*

Some people take this passage to mean that you can't tell anyone that you're fasting. I don't believe that to be true. You can tell people, but you should never show off. Don't behave like you're so weak from fasting and you're such a saint for doing it.

75

The Power of Fasting

There's a story I love about two men, one young and one older, who work for eight hours cutting down trees. The young guy chops down tree after tree and never stops for the entire day. The older man takes a break every hour for 15 minutes. The young man is proud and figures he will definitely beat the old man. However, at the end of the day the young man is surprised to see that the older man has chopped down more trees than him. He asks the old man how this is possible when he took so many breaks.

The old man replies, "I did take breaks, but when I did, I took time to sharpen my ax."

I believe fasting is a spiritual discipline that "sharpens your ax." You strengthen or "sharpen" your ability to take control of your body when you fast.

> ## Matthew 9:15 (NIV)
> *15 Jesus answered, "How can the guests of the bridegroom mourn while he is with them? The time will come when the bridegroom will be taken from them; then they will fast.*

Jesus made it clear that fasting would be a priority for us in His absence. We can't see Jesus and speak with Him face-to-face, but when we fast, it's like the next best thing. Fasting brings you as close as you can get to Him. It's a special bond between you and God.

76

Why Intermittent Fasting?

Intermittent fasting is exactly what it sounds like: it's alternating between eating and fasting for set periods of time. These periods of time are called **eating windows** and **fasting windows**. The secret sauce to the Chantel Ray Way has nothing to do with restricting what foods you can eat – in fact you can eat what you want. The secret sauce is reducing the number of hours a day you spend eating.

You have to understand that the human body wasn't meant to be scarfing down food non-stop throughout the day. In fact, you're going to learn about people who eat just once a day and are perfectly healthy and thin. Our biggest problem is overfeeding ourselves and intermittent fasting solves that problem.

There are new studies every day that continue to prove the benefits of intermittent fasting. The main reason that it's so effective for losing weight has everything to do with **insulin**. We're not going to get too scientific here, and I encourage you to do your own research to verify what I'm saying, but I want you to know that if you're someone who deals with diabetic issues, this plan can still be for you. I'm someone who at my highest weight was pre-diabetic, and I still have ongoing blood sugar issues. However, intermittent fasting has greatly impacted my blood sugar to the positive. If you have the same health issues I do, then you'll fit right in. Of course, consult your physician before starting a new diet plan.

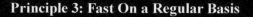

Principle 3: Fast On a Regular Basis

I check my blood sugar on a regular basis and I believe that's an important practice to begin. I've learned a lot about insulin and its role in regulating your body's glucose. When you eat, your blood sugar is available to either be burned as energy or stored as fat. In order to lose weight, you have to lower your insulin levels so that your body can access your stored fat effectively. The very act of eating, regardless of what you're eating, causes insulin to be released from your body. Fasting, on the other hand, lowers insulin which contributes to weight loss.

Anytime insulin increases, it can inhibit fat breakdown which is what you need for fat loss. Like I said before, anytime you eat, your insulin increases. How much it increases depends on several factors like the food and the person eating it, but now you should be able to see how fasting has a positive impact on fat loss. A scientific study actually revealed that the greatest drop in insulin and the greatest increase in fat breakdown take place between 18 and 24 hours of fasting.[3] Dr. Ted Naiman of burnfatnotsugar.com has a great graph that illustrates this. I've included it below with his permission:

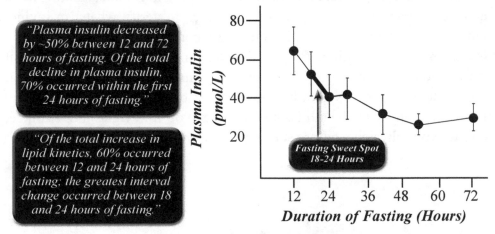

"Plasma insulin decreased by ~50% between 12 and 72 hours of fasting. Of the total decline in plasma insulin, 70% occurred within the first 24 hours of fasting."

"Of the total increase in lipid kinetics, 60% occurred between 12 and 24 hours of fasting; the greatest interval change occurred between 18 and 24 hours of fasting."

Fasting Sweet Spot 18-24 Hours

Duration of Fasting (Hours)

"These results demonstrate that the mobilization of adipose tissue triglycerides increases markedly between 18 and 24 hours of fasting."

Everything that we're talking about with intermittent fasting rides on insulin. You need your insulin to be low enough to promote fat breakdown so you can be in a fat-burning mode and not a sugar-burning mode.

[3] Progressive alterations in lipid and glucose metabolism during short-term fasting in young adult men S. Klein, Y. Sakurai, J. A. Romijn, R. M. Carroll American Journal of Physiology - Endocrinology and Metabolism Published 1 November 1993 Vol. 265 no. 5, E801-E806 DOI:

Principle 3: Fast On a Regular Basis

The Fasting Schedule

Now that you have a better understanding of intermittent fasting and its benefits, it's time to learn how to put it to work. The tables below detail the length of your eating windows and how many days a week you should be using that window to get you started. Notice that you can choose any day of the week that you like. Create your own schedule that works for you.

I recommend starting with an eight hour window. If you aren't losing weight as aggressively as you would like, move onto Phase 2.

Phase 1

Number Of Days Out Of The Week
Every day

Time Frame That You Can Eat Within
8 Hours

Phase 2

Number Of Days Out Of The Week
Every day

Time Frame That You Can Eat Within
6 Hours

All of the days in Phase 2 have six-hour eating windows. If you're eating for six hours, then you're fasting for 18. 18 hours of fasting gets you right into that fat burning zone you want to be in. In my experience, a six-hour or less eating window gets the best results. If you get comfortable with the six-hour window, you can step it up to Phase 3 and maximize your fat-burning.

79

Phase 3	Number Of Days Out Of The Week	Time Frame That You Can Eat Within
	4	6 Hours
	2	2 Hours
	1	8 Hours

I want to make a note about the four-hour eating window - also called the Big Power Fast. A four-hour window only gives you time to eat one meal for the day. This is essentially a 24-hour fast. Once you start your next window the following day, it will have been almost 24 hours since your last meal. I recommend doing the Big Power Fast on days when you know you're going to be very busy and not tempted to give in and break your fast.

Getting Too Hungry with the Big Power Fast

Years ago, my church participated in an eight-day corporate fast. It was the longest I had ever fasted and I kept up my regular exercise and work schedule. Because I didn't build up to it, I was ravenous by the end of the fast. Once it was over, I overate big time for the next five days and gained weight.

You may never find yourself fasting that long, but it is possible to let yourself get too hungry. This is the reason you should build up to the Big Power Fast. Like I've said before, fasting is like running. You don't go outside and run 10 miles when you've never run before, and you can't expect to do a 24 hour fast without some fasting experience. Take a measured approach to your fasting so you don't feel like you're starving and want to binge.

After you do a Big Power Fast, you **will** feel hungrier for the next couple of days. You're going to eat a little bit more because of that. However, if you get to the point that you're just shoveling it in, then it's better to stick to a six-hour eating window for a little bit longer. Day by day, start making that window smaller. Five hours one day, four hours the next, continuing until you reach your goal.

If you fast for 24 hours and then eat 3000 calories in one sitting, you're defeating the purpose of the fast. You're not to eat past a 4 on the hunger scale no matter what.

The Fed State vs The Fasted State

At any given time, your body is in one of two states: the **fed state** or the **fasted state**. Your body behaves very differently in both states. In the fed state, your body is actively digesting food and absorbing nutrients. How long it lasts depends on how long it takes for your body to digest food.

One of the factors that impact your digestion time is the kind of food you eat. Some foods digest faster than others and there's even a topic called **food combining** that explains how different foods digest better or worse when they're eaten together. I want to discuss food combining for just a minute because I did a popular food combining diet years ago. It made me crazy! The diet centered around eliminating, separating, or combining all kinds of different foods. I learned the hard way that it made me focus too much on what I was eating instead of how much I was eating. However, it wasn't all bad because I did learn a few things about my digestion. I learned that if I eat smaller portions, my body can digest most combinations of food. If I'm ravenously hungry and need to eat a little more, protein and vegetables digest together well for me.

The other state, the fasted state, technically begins when your body has finished digesting food. However, that's hard to track, so, for the purposes of this book, we're doing a tweaked version of the fasted state. When I mention being in a fasted state, I'm simply referring to the period of time after you closed your eating window. It's not technically accurate, but it's easier to track and it will work for the plan we're doing.

Getting to a true fasted state is something everyone should experience. The Big Power Fast allows you to do that with its one meal a day window. I believe that if you're constantly feeding your body and making it digest food pretty much 24/7, you're "hogging up" all of its time, so to speak. Your body never has a chance to renew itself. I believe fasting gives your body that opportunity and there's ongoing research to suggest intermittent fasting could help you live longer.

What Can I Eat While I'm Fasting?

While you're fasting, you are not to have any food whatsoever. The only things you can drink are liquids that don't have any calories. So, you can have black coffee, tea, water and sparkling unflavored water. Don't have any caloric drinks like diet soda or tea with stevia. You also can't pop mints, chew sugared gum, take cream in your coffee, or have a hard candy. There is no sugar whatsoever allowed on your fast! Whenever you have sugar – truthfully, whenever you eat anything at all - your insulin spikes. Spiking your insulin during your fast will lock away your fat stores and that's the opposite of what you want to happen. Accessing and burning that stored fat is a primary goal of fasting. Besides, if you're constantly eating little things during your fast you're going to counteract your ability to hear your body tell you when it's actually hungry.

It may sound obvious, but, when you're fasting, you're not eating. No exceptions. Some diet books talk about "free foods" – foods that have zero calories - as exceptions to the rule. Free foods can include diet Jello, pickles, carrots, plain celery, and more. Intermittent fasting, however, doesn't allow free foods, either.

Now, some people feel they can't survive without having *something* while they're fasting. They feel they have to have at least a diet soda or tea with stevia or something. If this is a real struggle for you, then I'd much rather you take baby steps and transition into full fasting. If you're one of those people, then you can start with **Crutch Foods** - we'll discuss this topic in detail in Principle 7 (on page 116). Crutch Foods technically break your fast, but you can start with them if going cold turkey is too hard. I'd rather you start there than not start at all.

Don't use this as an excuse to cheat on fasting! Know what you can handle, but don't be afraid to challenge yourself. It's a rewarding experience to be able to say "no" to food for a good chunk of your day. Don't rob yourself of that victory. You can do this!

82

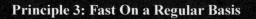

Do Not Overeat

Proverbs 25:16 (NIV)
[16] *If you find honey, eat just enough—too much of it, and you will vomit.*

Proverbs 23:21 (MSG)
Drunks and gluttons will end up on skid row, in a stupor and dressed in rags.

You have to stay on track with this one important aspect of intermittent fasting: it's all about not overeating. You can spend most of the day fasting, but if you gorge yourself on a ton of food when it's time to eat, you won't lose any weight. That's because you've eaten way more calories than you needed to. I want to make this very clear: do not overeat at any time!

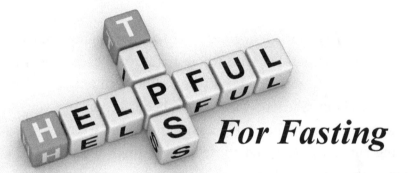

For Fasting

Build up to fasting. Intermittent fasting is the only diet that gets easier as you go. So, one thing you can do wrong in the beginning is fast for too long and binge. We know that in order to lose fat you have to have a caloric deficit, so if you binge you're going to ruin the whole point of fasting. If you fast too long in the beginning of this journey, it's going to make you very vulnerable to losing control and binge eating. It's better to start out slow. An eight-hour eating window is very, very easy to start with. While you should ultimately want to follow the schedule I laid out for you, it's okay to work your way there.

83

Stay busy. It really doesn't matter if you're playing video games, working, or reading a book. During your fasting time, especially when you start getting really hungry, you want to make sure you stay really, really busy. Sundays are a hard day for me because I'm more relaxed and that gives me room to eat. What I like to do is go to the mall and window shop, get my hair or nails done, or read God's word to stay busy.

Hunger comes in waves. When you're fasting, there's going to be a point when you get ravenously hungry, but after a little while it passes. No one stays starving for hours. Hunger comes in waves. If you can keep busy and pass that first couple of waves, you'll have more fat loss. People who are really thin are able to "ride that wave." It's just like a literal wave in the ocean that peaks up and then goes back down. Thin people understand that they can ride that out because they know the hunger will eventually go down.

Break your fast with whole, clean foods. You need to listen to what your body is wanting, but with whole foods. You can't feed your body a bunch of processed junk foods and then allow it to tell you what it wants. The chemicals in that food throw your body off making you want more and more junk food. When I'm breaking my fast, I try not to break it with anything but really clean and nutrient-dense foods. I definitely don't break my fast with chemicals. You also want to make sure that whatever your first meal is, it's not filled with sugar. Otherwise, you'll end up overeating.

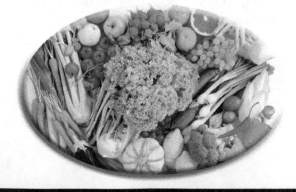

Use Potassium. I feel the best when I have plenty of potassium and without enough of it I feel I have no energy. My favorite sources of potassium are avocados, coconut water, bananas, and white potatoes. If you like avocados like I do, watch your intake. They're high in calories and you can consume a whole lot without even realizing it. The same goes for the sugar in coconut water.

Walk Away. Learn how to walk away from the food when you're done with it. It's okay to put away leftovers. When you know you can only eat once or twice a day you have a tendency to want to overeat. Make sure that you're eating foods that you actually like so you're not feeling deprived.

Get Extra Sleep. Sleep is very important. Your insulin decreases while you're sleeping and cortisol, which helps with blood sugar regulation, increases.

Get Active. I've taken to nightly walks with a friend. It's helping me lose weight and giving me something to do besides eat.

Drink Water. I drink a tall glass of water when I get really hungry. If that doesn't work, I'll have coffee with coconut oil or unsweetened tea.

Get Productive Early. I get annoyed if I eat before 12pm because I know I'm most productive in the morning when I haven't eaten yet. After eating, my productivity drops. Try to prolong your fasting window so that you can be more productive. See if you can push yourself one more hour even when you think you can't.

Find a Friend. Find a friend you can do intermittent fasting with so you can hold each other accountable.

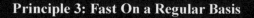

85

Eat More Protein. Getting more protein in your diet leads to greater appetite control. Find a way to get it in while still eating what you want.

Read The Bible. Draw strength from scriptures. The Bible tells us to fast, so it's something we know we can do.

Remember It Doesn't Happen Overnight. One thing you have to remember when you start this plan is that you're not going to lose weight as fast as you want to. I personally didn't lose any weight for the first two weeks. This plan has to be looked at over the course of a month. On my third week, I lost 6lbs. My fourth week, 4lbs. Intermittent fasting is not a get skinny quick scheme. It's not overnight, but that's okay because you want this to be lasting. You didn't gain the weight overnight, and you can't lose it overnight. We are making a lifestyle change that's forever. In the book of Exodus, you can read about the Israelites' trials in the desert. There are going to be times when you feel like you're in the desert and aren't losing weight. The thing with this diet is, you'll lose fat, but not muscle. So, there will be some weeks when you feel like you aren't losing weight. But instead of feeling miserable like you're in the desert and depriving yourself, take it as an opportunity to ask God, "What are You going to show me today? What are You going to teach me?"

Another tip is to save your coffee for later in your fast, not first thing in the morning. If you choose to set your fast for the morning hours, you'll notice that you're usually not hungry when you first wake up. That's one of the reasons I prefer morning fasts. There's a myth out there that breakfast is the most important meal of the day, but it's simply not true. You can choose to fast whenever you like and get results. You're already in a fasted state when you first wake up in the morning, so save your coffee for when your hunger starts to creep up so the caffeine can suppress your appetite.

Fasting: It Works!

There are benefits to intermittent fasting that I haven't found with any diet I've tried. First, I believe intermittent fasting is a solution for the "willpower factor." I think we all have a limit to our willpower. We can get excited about a diet for a little while, but, when we want a brownie and the diet says we can't, most times we end up failing. We move on to the next diet since the last one was "too hard" and when that one fails we move on to another one. We blame the diets, but it's really our inability to stick with them that's the problem - but that's okay! Trying to live by a diet is unrealistic and unsustainable. Diets that restrict foods get harder the longer you do them while intermittent fasting is the only plan that I believe gets easier with time. It doesn't put pressure on your willpower because you're still allowed to eat what you want. You're simply changing the time frame that you eat in.

The second major benefit is that I'm finally eating less. I'm at the point where I'm eating only two meals just about every day, and they're small meals at that. See, my struggles with eating are just like my troubles with skiing. I do great while I'm in motion, but I'm atrocious at stopping. They had to stamp a big, red "X" on my ticket and threaten to kick me off the slope if I didn't stop running into people! Well, stopping once I start eating is just as real a challenge for me. Intermittent fasting has helped me control and stop my eating when I need to.

Now, I'm even snacking less. I literally had a snacking addiction to the point where my family made up a song to tease me: it's called "All I Do is Snack" to the tune of "All I Do is Win" by DJ Khaled. Yes, it was that bad. Thankfully, my snacking addiction is broken now, and you won't find me snacking all day anymore.

Finally, when it comes to my health, my hormones feel regulated, my immune system is stronger, and I have more mental clarity. There are so many different cleanses out there, but I believe fasting is God's way of doing it. It's like a self-cleansing process. Don't waste your money on cleanses when you can just fast. Your body gets a chance to repair itself while you fast. Fasting works!

Alternative Intermittent Fasting Methods

If you've never heard of intermittent fasting before now, you're probably going to Google it to learn more. When you do, you'll find out there are a lot of different versions and suggestions about how to do it.

Here are a few that I've seen but don't recommend that you follow.

5-2 Diet. This diet involves eating a normal, healthy diet five days of the week, and then eating only 500 calories for two days of the week. Those days would be your fast days. My problem with this diet is that I believe it requires too much calorie counting and could ultimately leave room for you to be tempted to binge.

Heavy Eating. There's a myth that you should eat a ton of food at your meals in your eating window to avoid snacking in between. I disagree because that would require you to overeat.

Early Dinners. There's a commonly held belief, whether you're doing intermittent fasting or not, that you should never eat dinner late at night. I have a ton of friends who have late eating windows and even eat carbs right before bed, and they're still very thin.

88

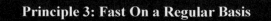

Closing Thoughts

I have a friend named Alison who has to be extremely strict when she's dieting because, if she ever slips, the whole thing goes down the drain. Are you that kind of person? Do you feel like if you indulge yourself even a little you're going to lose control? Well consider what I said before about diets not being sustainable. Think about it: even when you were on your strictest diet, did you stick to it in the end? So, what was the point of denying yourself the foods you like if the diet wasn't sustainable anyway?

When I was getting married, I wanted to lose a bunch of weight to be really skinny for my wedding dress. So, for 30 days all I had was a protein shake for breakfast, and chicken and broccoli for lunch and dinner. I lost 15lbs in those 30 days and dropped from a dress size 8 to a 4. However, on my honeymoon I gained seven pounds in seven days! See my point?

Intermittent fasting with the Chantel Ray Way is different. It's meant to be something that lasts. As you continue reading, you'll learn that there are no restrictions on eating the things that you want; that's something you don't have to be afraid of! You're going to learn how to eat intuitively. You're going to learn how to listen to your body, eat only when you're hungry, and stop when you're full. This plan isn't going to restrict you. It's going to give you back control over your food like you've never had before. You're not going to have to plan all of your meals and worry about whether the party you're going to has food that fits in your diet.

Principle 4: *Limit Sugar Intake*

Proverbs 25:27 (NLT)
27 It's not good to eat too much honey, and it's not good to seek honors for yourself.

In Principle 3, we talked a little bit about insulin and blood sugar, but now we'll tackle the topic with sugar in more detail so you can understand the importance of avoiding too much sugar in your diet.

Sugar-Burning vs Fat-Burning

It's very important that you understand the two modes your body can be in at any given time: **fat-burning** or **sugar-burning**. You have to be in a fat-burning state to lose weight. The ultimate goal is to create a system of eating where you're consistently in a fat-burning state without cutting all sugar out of your diet.

As soon as you eat food, the storage hormone called insulin starts to rise. It signals the cells in your body to absorb glucose. When we stop eating, insulin levels fall and after so many hours of fasting we use up all the sugar and switch over to fat for fuel-burning. This is similar to why you don't have to eat while you're asleep. Your body is using stored energy to survive.

Think of a hybrid car. Some hybrids use only electricity for fuel until there's none left. At that point, it switches over to gas consumption to keep going. That is what it's like in the human body. You want to use up all that sugar and get to the fat because burning fat results in weight loss.

90

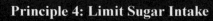

Your body won't bother going to fat stores for fuel when there's plenty of sugar present. When you start your fast, your body is burning only sugar at first. After 18-24 hours those stores start to run out, so your body is forced to get energy from your fat. That's the key! Now you know why low-carb high-fat diets work so well. There's less sugar for your body to pull from when you're eating that way. Like all diets, though, it's hard to sustain so we want to find a way to have balance.

Blood Sugar

An ideal blood sugar level is between 80-100 while you're fasting. I feel the best when my blood sugar is between 80-100 while I'm fasting. If I'm starting to fall into a slump, I use exercise or caffeine to perk me up. Since you shouldn't be consuming calories during your fasting window, you can drink unsweetened tea or black coffee to get your caffeine.

Your body gets its fuel from three kinds of food: carbohydrates, proteins, and fats. Carbohydrates (carbs) come from breads, fruits, vegetables and more. Fat and protein come from dairy, nuts, and fatty vegetables like avocados. Your digestive system breaks down each food and basically sends it to your blood stream. Your body uses insulin to process the sugar from the carbs you eat. So, the amount of insulin your body creates really depends on how much sugar you're taking in. When you hear the word "sugar" you might be visualizing table sugar, but sugar also comes from the breakdown of carbs.

When I eat a meal that's high in sugar, I immediately crave a snack afterwards. It's not that I'm still hungry; I just feel the need for something sweet. This is because the high-sugar meal I ate caused my blood sugar to shoot up high. So, when that blood sugar drops even just a little, I start craving something sweet to balance me out. This is a major reason to avoid eating too much sugar.

91

Glycemic Index/Glycemic Load

A lot of the diets you've tried pushed the rule of restricting carbs to lose weight, but not all carbs are created equal. 50g of carbs from bread and 50g of carbs from broccoli don't release the same amount of sugar into your bloodstream. These differences in foods can be determined by the **glycemic index** or **glycemic load** of a particular food. There is a difference between those two terms, but they both are used to determine what effect the food you eat has on your blood sugar.

Should you spend a lot of time obsessing over the glycemic load of the foods you eat? No, not at all. I don't think there are thin people out there calculating the glycemic load of two cups of spaghetti versus corn on the cob. That sort of stressful calculation will drive you crazy just like dieting. That being said, I do think you should be conscious of the amount of sugar you're eating. All of the thin eaters I talked to really watched the amount of sugar they consumed. I consciously keep my diet with 80% of foods that don't drastically raise my blood sugar. It's not hard to see that an apple isn't going to raise your blood sugar the same way a donut will, right? Keep your blood sugar under control or it's going to make you want to keep eating more.

Monitoring Your Blood Sugar

Oftentimes, people will try to rid their diets of all sugar. That's unrealistic for me, so I focus on tracking my blood sugar level. One option to monitor your blood sugar is a **continuous glucose monitor (CGM).** A CGM shows you your blood sugar level minute by minute, but it's very expensive. It costs about $300 to lease for two weeks or $1800 to buy outright, and you have to have a prescription notice from your physician. Instead, I recommend you use something like the Freestyle Lite blood glucose monitor. Using the Freestyle Lite, I learned a lot about my body that I didn't know before. For example, if I have a cup of coffee with coconut oil, it literally reduces my blood sugar by 10-15 points. So, if I'm fasting and my blood sugar is 85, after a cup of coffee with a heaping tablespoon of coconut oil, I end up at 75. However, I feel energized, not hypoglycemic.

The Freestyle Lite makes small and almost painless pin pricks. I got it for only $19 at Walgreens without a prescription. You can order 50 test strips for it from Amazon for $26.

92

Your Blood Sugar Report Card

Once you have the ability to check your blood sugar on a regular basis, you have to know where your blood sugar should be. I asked my stepfather, who is a doctor, to help me create a report card to measure how I'm doing. When you're in the discovery phase, take your blood sugar 3 or 4 times a day to learn your levels and responses. Later, you won't have to test it so much.

GRADE	Blood Sugar While Fasting	Blood Sugar After Eating
A	70-90	100 or less
B	91-100	101-110
C	101-110	111-120
D	111+	121+

Personally, the pounds shed right off when I stay consistently below 100. Check your sugar 30 minutes after you eat and then again 2 hours after. The second reading will be most accurate.

Being accountable with my blood sugar helped me decide how many grams of sugar to eat per day. I like to have only 20. It may be different for you, so start getting acquainted with your blood sugar and find out what works for you.

**For more information on blood sugar,
go to: www.ChantelRayWay.com/bloodsugar**

93

Principle 5:
Don't Make Food Your Idol

The Idol
of Food

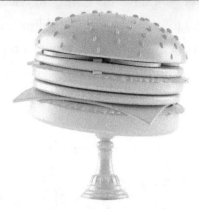

Exodus 34:14 (NLT)
You must worship no other gods, for the Lord, whose very name is Jealous, is a God who is jealous about his relationship with you.

You may be wondering what idol worship has to do with weight loss. When we hear the word "idol" we think of it as Exodus 20 describes it.

Exodus 20:1-6 (MSG)
God spoke all these words:
I am God, your God,
who brought you out of the land of Egypt,
out of a life of slavery.
No other gods, only me.
No carved gods of any size, shape, or form of anything
whatever, whether of things that fly or walk or swim.
Don't bow down to them and don't serve them because
I am God, your God...

However, an idol can be more than just a carved object. An idol is **anything we place in a position of worship over God or His commandments**. I believe one of the chief idols in America today is **food**. Most Americans are in love with food - heart, mind, and soul.

94

"That's not true," you might say. "Food isn't my idol. I'm just overweight because I'm eating the wrong food and I don't exercise enough."

That is just not the case! It's your being in love with food that's the problem. Think about what it's like when you first fall in love with someone. I remember what it was like when I first started dating my husband, Rhyan. I always had my nails and hair done and I had to have the perfect outfit when I knew I was going to see him. He was all I thought about. When you're in love, the object of your affection is the number one thing on your mind and every plan you make revolves around it. That's what I see happening with people and food. We're not even done with breakfast and we're thinking about what's for lunch. If there's no good food at a party, then we don't want to be there. A wedding with bad food is considered a bad wedding. EVERYTHING revolves around food.

This obsession with food usually starts in childhood. Growing up, food was given to me as a reward for good behavior. These are things I try to do differently with my son. I don't tell him that he won't get any ice cream if he doesn't finish everything on his dinner plate. These kinds of statements seem innocent at first, but they become ingrained in us and shape how we look at food when we get older.

If you want to find out what a person loves, see what they focus on the most. One of the things I love the most are my kids. So much of what my husband and I talk, think, and plan about are them. Think for a second: how much of your daily conversation is about food? How much do you think about it? Are you constantly counting calories? How many of your social activities are scheduled around your eating? Once again, this is why I'm so against diets. As a dieter you have to constantly read labels, count every little calorie, read every book on what to eat and what not to eat. It's a never-ending cycle of obsession.

> **Exodus 32:2-4 (MSG)**
> *So, Aaron told them, "Take off the gold rings from the ears of your wives and sons and daughters and bring them to me." They all did it; they removed the gold rings from their ears and brought them to Aaron. He took the gold from their hands and cast it in the form of a calf, shaping it with an engraving tool.*
> *The people responded with enthusiasm: "These are your gods, O Israel, who brought you up from Egypt!"*

In times past, when I read this story about the Israelites worshiping the golden calf, I always said, "What is wrong with these people? Are they really that stupid that they would make this golden calf themselves and then bow down to it?" But if you think about it, that is what we're doing with food and it's almost worse. We're bowing down to a piece of pizza or an ice cream cone.

It's weird for us because none of us make a gold calf and worship it, but we have our own false god that we turn to for comfort. If you're reading this book, it probably means that you made food your false god.

> **Isaiah 44:9 (NLT)**
> [9] *How foolish are those who manufacture idols. These prized objects are really worthless. The people who worship idols don't know this, so they are all put to shame.*

When I was in my 20's, I noticed all of my thin friends were eating candy and junk food and staying thin. I ate grilled chicken and broccoli and couldn't lose a pound. Because I wanted to be like them I ended up in a bulimic lifestyle. I ate whatever I wanted and threw it up later. At this point in my life, I was obsessed with food. Every decision was between being thin or eating what I wanted and purging later. I used laxatives, water pills, and exercised compulsively. I knew I was in bondage and I was scared it would last forever. Finally, I prayed and declared that no matter what I ate, I wasn't going to throw up again. God answered and delivered me.

Now, I recognize that food had become my idol during that season of my life. It was something I worshiped and it dominated my every decision. You can be vegan if you want to be vegan and you can eat paleo if you want to eat paleo. What you should never do is be in bondage. Analyzing every label, counting every calorie, and measuring every meal is stressful and it's idolatry.

We were all born to worship something and God put a worship pacemaker in each and every one of our hearts. If we don't know God to worship Him, then there's a God-shaped hole in our hearts that we try to fill with other things. It can be food, sex, money, drugs, work, or just about anything. This is what idolatry is. It used to be statues and animal heads, but now it's these subtle things we make our obsessions.

When you idolize these other things, it's like committing spiritual adultery. Striving to be healthy is good, but when you become obsessive and set that pursuit ahead of God then there's an issue. You can't love something God made more than you love Him and no one can serve two masters (Matthew 6:24). We never set out to make idols out of our diets. However, if you're living life scared to eat and you're up all night feeling guilty about what you *did* eat, then that's exactly what you've done.

Intermittent fasting has helped me take charge and overcome all of this craziness. Pray and ask the Holy Spirit to grant you wisdom to make good choices and be balanced.

1 Corinthians 3:16 (NIV)

16 Don't you know that you yourselves are God's temple and that God's Spirit dwells in your midst?

If I were in someone else's house, I would be very careful with everything. Remember that your body doesn't belong to you. It belongs to God!

God's ways are always better. You're going to have a desert experience of testing where you have to decide whether or not you're going to do it His way. When you do it His way, He'll come in and reward you.

Recently, I went to Chipotle with my family. Everyone ordered food but my stomach wasn't growling so I ordered a side of chicken to take home. 30 minutes after I got home, I was hungry. My food was still warm, so I ate and felt rewarded for making the right decision.

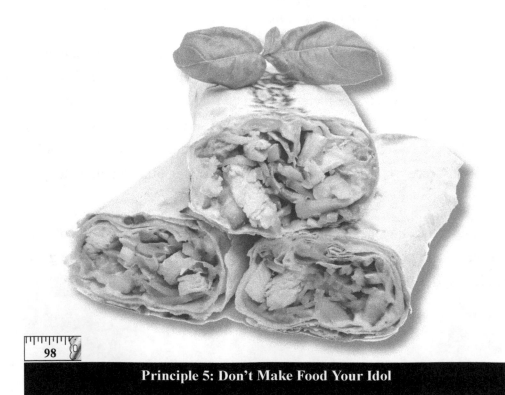

Principle 5: Don't Make Food Your Idol

The Three Signs of Worship

I believe there are three major signs of worship that can be identified in every person. When you worship something, there are three things that you do.

1. FOCUS ON IT

Hebrews 12:2 (NIV)
Fixing our eyes on Jesus, the pioneer and perfecter of faith. For the joy set before him he endured the cross, scorning its shame, and sat down at the right hand of the throne of God.

Our focus is meant to be on Jesus, but when we become fixated on diets and losing weight to the point of obsession we are out of focus.

Romans 12:1 (NIV)
Therefore, I urge you, brothers and sisters, in view of God's mercy, to offer your bodies as a living sacrifice, holy and pleasing to God—this is your true and proper worship.

2. GIVE YOURSELF TO IT

We're meant to give ourselves to God, not to donuts! It sounds almost silly, but how many times have we surrendered our wills to the desire for food?

3. FIND JOY IN IT

Psalm 16:11 (NIV)
You make known to me the path of life; you will fill me with joy in your presence, with eternal pleasures at your right hand.

While I believe God means for us to enjoy the food we eat, food was never meant to be the *source* of our joy.

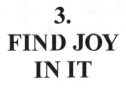

99

The Fear of Food

I finally lost the obsession of what to eat when I began intermittent fasting. I finally lost the weight even though I wasn't eating perfect with every single meal. I lost the fear of food that dominated every diet that I ever tried.

When I was growing up in school I was taught about the food pyramid. The way I remember it, there were basically four categories of food: dairy, grains, fruits and vegetables, and meat. Do a web search today on any of those food groups and here's some of the things you'll see people saying about them.

Dairy:
THE MEDIA SAYS: Dairy is SO bad for you! Cow's milk is only meant for baby cows and humans should never drink it. Dairy products have no place in your diet. Period!

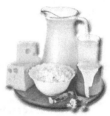

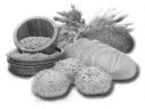

Grains and Bread:
THE MEDIA SAYS: Grains are killing you as you speak! They can destroy your intestinal tract and gluten has detrimental effects on your brain. Grain is poison.

Fruits and Vegetables:
THE MEDIA SAYS: There's a whole group of vegetables called nightshade vegetables that includes potatoes, tomatoes, eggplants, bell peppers and more. These vegetables are deadly and include over 2,000 different species.

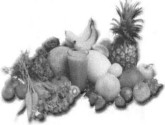

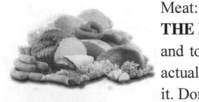

Meat:
THE MEDIA SAYS: Red meat has too much fat and too many calories. Fish is good, but then it actually isn't because it has too much mercury in it. Don't eat poultry because it has salmonella.

You can find dozens of articles condemning every possible food you can think of including water! It's gotten to the point that you don't know what to eat or drink anymore. There's always a new fad and dieting trend to chase. Tell me you haven't seen these headlines before:

"Top 10 Superfoods to Keep in Your Kitchen!"

"3 Foods to Make You Lose Weight Right Away!"

"Eat These Foods to Lose Belly Fat Fast!

This culture of fearing food is a form of idol worship sustained by the media, self-proclaimed diet gurus, and even doctors.

Food is Not the Problem

There are a lot of people that view food as the source of their problems. They decide to eat nothing but celery and carrots and ban wheat and eggs and just restrict, restrict, restrict. As a result, they still end up eating large portions of whatever it is they do allow themselves to eat.

> ### 1 Corinthians 10:31 (NIV)
> *31 So whether you eat or drink or whatever you do, do it all for the glory of God.*

> ### Colossians 2:20-22 (NASB)
> *20 ...why, as if you were living in the world, do you submit yourself to decrees, such as, 21 "Do not handle, do not taste, do not touch!" 22 (which all refer to things destined to perish with use)...*

In my opinion, there is nothing in the Bible that tells you that you can't eat this or that.

101

Binging

Exodus 34:14 (NLT)
14 You must worship no other gods, for the Lord, whose very name is Jealous, is a God who is jealous about his relationship with you.

I went to college for a degree in math and during that time I was under extreme amounts of stress. In fact, my third and fourth years of college were the most stressful times in my life. In high school, I made straight A's and never studied. I never had to work hard at anything. But then I went to Virginia Wesleyan University because I wanted to be a math teacher. Your first two years of math are reasonable. It's when you become a math major that you get to the point where you aren't even dealing with numbers anymore. It gets out there! It was so far beyond me that I felt like I didn't even know what I was doing.

All of this stress drove me into bulimia. I would literally binge eat and then throw up because I didn't want to gain too much weight. I had all of this anxiety, and I would just eat, eat, eat, and get myself to the point where I was so sick I would force myself to throw up. For two years I was this way - binging and purging repeatedly. It was a really bad time for me. When I wasn't throwing up I was using laxatives. I was going to the gym and I would work out for 2-3 hours a day. I was just consumed with worry about my weight. It was really just a horrible, stressful time in my life.

If any of this sounds like your life and if you're struggling with bulimia then here's something you need to do:

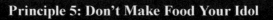

1. First of all, repent and ask God for help. I had to recognize that I had a food addiction and needed to set boundaries. I could never binge. I could never overeat.

2. Stop depriving yourself through dieting. The reason why people purge like this is because they are dieting so much. During my struggle, I was telling myself "I am only going to eat broccoli and cucumbers and carrots and grilled chicken." You can only do that for so long. Because I was depriving myself, the second I got in contact with a donut I couldn't just eat half of it. I had to eat 10 because I hadn't had anything sweet in two weeks.

3. Every time you feel like you're going to overeat or binge, spend that time with God. You have to go to God and ask for help when you're tempted to bypass the boundaries you set for yourself. Ask Him to fill you up better than food ever could. Instead of binging on food you're saying "God, can you do better than the binge?"

4. Know that there is no deprivation. Tell yourself, "I am not depriving myself of anything. If there is anything I want to eat, I may eat it. I am going to make wise choices and I'm not going to eat everything at once. If I want half of a donut, I can have half of a donut. I'm not going to be afraid of eating certain things."

You DON'T have forbidden fruits. As soon as something is a forbidden fruit in your mind, you crave it. There is no forbidden fruit in this lifestyle. There is nothing you can't eat. You are re-introducing yourself to food and you are CHOOSING to eat healthy foods much of the time. I eat a little bit of something that would be considered "off-limits" on a traditional diet every day.

There is almost a sense of peace when you get hungry and it's in that time frame where you know you can eat again. If you listen to your body, it will tell you what you want to eat. My favorite treat used to be Twizzlers, but, at one time, everyone was giving me all of these Twizzlers, so for a couple of weeks I couldn't even eat a Twizzler! I had had too much and my body knew it.

You don't have to try to completely ignore your cravings. If you're craving salt, don't buy unsalted chips. If you're craving salt you probably need it for whatever reason. You just want to remember to rate your foods and only eat what you really want. If someone brought in blueberry muffins and someone else brought in Krispy Kreme donuts, I would want the muffin. However, I would only eat the muffin top because that's my highest rated thing. Just eat the best things!

Why Man-Made Diets Fail

I tried every diet known to man and they gave me more issues with food than I had before.

> ### Colossians 2:20-23 (NIV)
> [20] *Since you died with Christ to the elemental spiritual forces of this world, why, as though you still belonged to the world, do you submit to its rules:* [21] *"Do not handle! Do not taste! Do not touch!"?* [22] *These rules, which have to do with things that are all destined to perish with use, are based on merely human commands and teachings.* [23] *Such regulations indeed have an appearance of wisdom, with their self-imposed worship, their false humility and their harsh treatment of the body, but they lack any value in restraining sensual indulgence.*

I kept reading all of these diet books instead of going to the Bible to find out what God said. When I went to the Word, I found out God had so much to say about fasting! I'm anti-diet because diets force you to focus more on food. They make a big greed problem because instead of addressing the problem of overeating they encourage you to have larger amounts of food. They justify it by labeling some foods as "good" and others as "bad." Instead of making us change our behavior, diets try to make the food behave. So we go after chemicals, artificial sugars, and all of this low-calorie fluff! We create habits of eating more food instead of waiting until we're hungry.

You can even lose weight on some of these diets even though you're overeating, but the Bible instructs us to refrain from gluttony. It doesn't say anything about low calorie foods being an exception. Diets also put you in a position where you're almost worshipping food because it becomes such a focus. Thin eaters don't focus on food that much. Thin eaters can even forget to eat.

These diets don't last because, at some point, you will go back to the foods you really want. This is because you never addressed the main issue: overeating. You never learned to listen to your hunger and fullness.

Acts 3:1 (NIV)
19 Repent, then, and turn to God, so that your sins may be wiped out, that times of refreshing may come from the Lord,

Repentance

Hebrews 3:7-11 (MSG)
*Today, please listen;
don't turn a deaf ear as in "the bitter uprising,"
that time of wilderness testing!
Even though they watched me at work for forty years,
our ancestors refused to let me do it my way;
over and over they tried my patience.
And I was provoked, oh, so provoked!
I said, "They'll never keep their minds on God;
they refuse to walk down my road."
Exasperated, I vowed,
"They'll never get where they're going,
never be able to sit down and rest."*

Repentance is easily defined as "turning from your old ways." It's something the Bible talks about often and it's very important. True repentance means doing a 180-degree turn. It's turning away from sin and turning back to God. It's loving Him and making Him who you turn to instead of food.

Ecclesiastes 6:7 (NIV)

⁷ Everyone's toil is for their mouth, yet their appetite is never satisfied.

Joel 2:26 (NIV)

²⁶ You will have plenty to eat, until you are full, and you will praise the name of the Lord your God, who has worked wonders for you; never again will my people be shamed.

I used to live for food. I planned my entire day around eating. I overindulged myself at breakfast while getting excited about lunch. I finally realized that my desire for food could never be satisfied because in a couple of hours I was going to want something else. The Chantel Ray Way keeps your mind off of eating and forces you to turn to God when you're hungry instead of turning to food.

Joel 2:12-13 (NASB)

¹² "Yet even now," declares the Lord,
"Return to Me with all your heart,
And with fasting, weeping and mourning;
¹³ And rend your heart and not your garments."
Now return to the Lord your God,
For He is gracious and compassionate,
Slow to anger, abounding in lovingkindness
And relenting of evil.

This goes back to acknowledging that overeating is a sin. As long as you're pretending that gluttony is fine, you're never going to repent and turn away from your behavior.

107

1 Corinthians 10:31 (NIV)
31 So whether you eat or drink or whatever you do, do it all for the glory of God.

1 Corinthians 3:17b (NLT)
...For God's temple is holy, and you are that temple.

Understand that when you commit the sin of gluttony you're harming your body, God's temple.

John 8:34 (NIV)
34 Jesus replied, "Very truly I tell you, everyone who sins is a slave to sin.

Sin leads to slavery. Overeating, just like any other sin, can be addictive. You become a slave to your own habits. It's a vicious cycle because the more you overeat, the more you want to overeat.

When someone is truly repentant, they're sorrowful for what they've done and they're not pointing the finger at somebody else. Many of us constantly blame others when it comes to our weight.

We say, "It's my husband's fault that I'm fat because he always brings junk food into the house." Or, "I blame my kids because they don't eat their half of the food."

That's not what real repentance looks like. Real repentance says, "I, and I alone, am the reason that I'm overweight."

It's not because your job is stressful or because your husband is mean to you. All of these crazy things people come up with are just excuses to overeat. This journey can only begin once you finally stop passing blame.

Hebrews 3:15 (NIV)
15 As has just been said: "Today, if you hear his voice, do not harden your hearts as you did in the rebellion."

Romans 12:1-2 (NIV)

[12] *Therefore, I urge you, brothers and sisters, in view of God's mercy, to offer your bodies as a living sacrifice, holy and pleasing to God—this is your true and proper worship. 2 Do not conform to the pattern of this world, but be transformed by the renewing of your mind. Then you will be able to test and approve what God's will is—his good, pleasing and perfect will.*

The 80/20 Rule

Because of my autoimmune disease (I'll discuss this in more detail later), I feel my absolute best when I'm eating clean – for me, that's a diet of meats (poultry, beef and seafood), fruits, non-starchy vegetables, nuts and seeds, and natural oils (olive oil, palm oil, etc.). I don't eat a lot of grains, dairy, beans, refined sugar, or processed oils like canola oil, vegetable oil, or soybean oil. This is **80%** of my diet, the other **20%** is whatever I want.

I didn't come by this mathematically. How I eat boils down to "how do I feel?" For example, last week my diet was probably more 60/40 and I can tell that I'm feeling tired and sluggish now because of it. This week, I'm back on track and feeling much better because of it.

109

The question you're going to ask is, "why not eat clean 100% of the time?" I know that if I did that I would feel absolutely FANTASTIC! But I also know that if I go down that road I'm going to go crazy. Trying to eat "perfect" is what made me obsessed with dieting. That's something you have to avoid. Eating 20% "non-clean" foods is enough that I don't feel deprived and not so much that my body is suffering because of it.

I am very against diets that deprive you of food because they leave you feeling overwhelmed. A 2011 New York Times study on "decision fatigue" discovered that prisoners who appeared before a particular parole board in the morning received parole 70% of the time. In the afternoon that number dropped to 10%[4]. I think the decision makers on that parole board heard one excuse after another and just got tired. It's what's called "decision fatigue." We as human beings get overwhelmed when we have too much information coming at us. There's no truer instance than when you're searching for the right diet. One book says "Food A leads to cancer and you should never eat it under any circumstances! But eat lots of Food B." However, the second book tears down Food B and champions Food A as the healthiest food in the world! Does that sound familiar?

Instead of driving myself crazy with diets that changed with the direction of the wind, I decided to focus on eating whole foods and as few chemicals as possible. I didn't ban the foods that I liked; I just made it my mission to find a way to satisfy my cravings without taking a trip to Chemical City.

[2] Tierny, John, "Do You Suffer From Decision Fatigue"
http://www.nytimes.com/2011/08/21/magazine/do-you-suffer-from-decision-fatigue.html

Chemical City

"Chemical City" is a phrase I use around my home to describe foods that I think are loaded with chemicals and are way unhealthy for you. If my son asks for something that I think crosses that line, my response is, "No way! That's Chemical City!" These are the foods I actively avoid. Let's take a look at your average coffee creamer for example:

Coffee creamer. The coffee creamer you have in your refrigerator or cabinet could be full of corn syrup solids and something called diglycerides. Diglyccrides alone can contain trans fats even if the nutrition label says there are no trans fats. Instead of coffee creamer, I'll use coconut milk if I absolutely need something extra in my coffee.

If I want a boost of energy, I'll have a green juice instead of an energy drink. Some of the ingredients found in energy drinks include sucralose and acesulfame potassium. Green juice is a much healthier option. I make mine with spinach, celery, kale, lemon, cucumber, and ginger.

A little side note about green juice: I think it's GREAT! If you're someone who doesn't like it, just give it a chance. Green juice replenishes you with vital nutrients and vitamins and counteracts cravings.

I use a Breville brand juicer for my green juice. It's a **masticating juicer** which is the most efficient kind. The other most popular option is a **centrifugal juicer**. This type of juicer is usually cheaper but not as effective at extracting all of the nutrients you want from fruits and vegetables.

Now, I think this goes without saying, but when I'm talking about juice in this section I am NOT referring to pasteurized juices you can buy from the store.

Another drink to mention when discussing chemicals is wine. We discuss wine in detail in this book, but, in short, I'm not against it if you can find an organic wine. If I drink two glasses of wine with chemicals in it I feel terrible the next day. The #1 chemical you can find in wine is **sulfur dioxide**. It can cause migraine headaches, skin irritations, breathing problems, and more. On top of that, wine has a lot of added sugar and pesticides are sprayed all over the grapes that make it. The workers who spray pesticide wear protective clothing like hazmat suits. Shouldn't that be a major red flag? If you drink organic red wine, you can avoid the pesticides. Visit ChantelRayWay.com to see what brands of wine I recommend along with some of my other favorite products.

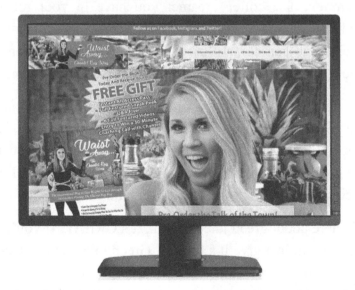

On the topic of alcohol, I need to state that I am anti-beer. Besides the fact that I can't stand the taste, beer is full of chemicals. Most beers are filled with high fructose corn syrups (HFCS), a lot of artificial flavors, and carrageenan.

> **1 Corinthians 6:19-20 (NIV)**
> *[19] Do you not know that your bodies are temples of the Holy Spirit, who is in you, whom you have received from God? You are not your own; [20] you were bought at a price. Therefore honor God with your bodies.*

In whatever you eat, remember that your body is a temple. If it's a temple, why would you put chemicals in it?

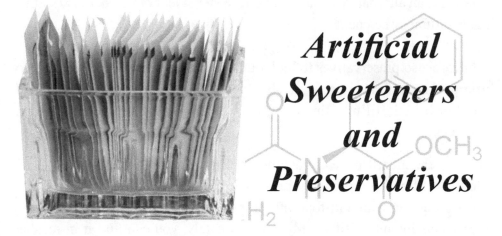

Artificial Sweeteners and Preservatives

I'm big on not drinking my calories, but I have a ton of super thin friends who do. For them, it comes mostly from wines and mixed drinks. If you keep it in your eating window, that's fine. However, I recommend staying far, far away from sodas. If you take 10 teaspoons of sugar and lay it on a table, you're looking at the amount of sugar in a 12oz can of soda. That's ridiculous! On top of that, it's not even real sugar! You're drinking something called high-fructose corn syrup (HFCS). It's a chemical derivative of corn syrup and you can find it in bread, yogurt, crackers, cookies, and more. HFCS is not real sugar. It's basically just straight chemicals. Now, I'm not anti-sugar. I just recommend real sugar. Raw sugar, raw honey, coconut sugar, dates, and maple sugar are all great options, but I avoid HFCS like the plague.

If you're on the lookout for artificial sweeteners, check the backs of the packaging on the foods you eat and look for these kinds of ingredients:

- **aspartame**
- **saccharin**
- **sucralose**
- **acesulfame potassium (acesulfame K)**

I prefer that you use real sugar rather than these ingredients or any artificial sugars. As an alternative to sugar, I believe stevia leaf or powder is OK since it is a natural sweetener.

There are also preservatives to look out for. For this reason, I try to eat very little packaged food. I prefer fresh foods as opposed to anything canned, jarred or boxed. If I'm eating corn, I want corn on the cob instead of corn from a can.

Another chemical I'm really against is **dimethylpolysiloxane**. Yes, that's a long word and it's probably present in a lot of the food you eat. It's a type of **silicone** with anti-foaming properties that's used in a wide variety of products including silly putty. Unfortunately, you can find it in mashed potatoes, and most fast food chicken sandwiches and french fries.

Azodicarbonamide, also called the "yoga mat compound," can be found in commercially baked bread. It's in almost 500 food products! As you could guess from the nickname, it's used in yoga mats and it's added to bread to maintain "texture." It's an unnecessary chemical.

You even have to watch out for the "healthy foods." You can find a chemical called carrageenan in almond milk. It's basically a thickener that keeps liquids from separating. It's allowed in organic foods and it's been linked to colon cancer, IBS, and gastrointestinal problems. I've started making my own almond milk because I haven't found any that doesn't have loads of chemicals in it.

114

Just about everyone knows about MSG, or, monosodium glutamate. It's in everything from restaurant foods to chips and frozen dinners.

If I look at a food label and I don't know what one of the ingredients is, then that's something I'm going to try to keep out of my diet. Take a look at the nutrition labels on the foods you eat every day and see what you find. Here are a few common foods and snacks and the suspicious ingredients you can find in them. It's eye-opening what you'll discover from a quick web search:

Deli Turkey Breast.
Contains carrageenan.

Cheese-flavored Nachos.
Contain MSG, corn syrup solids and artificial colors like Yellow 6 or Red 40.

Cereal Bars.
Contain high fructose corn syrup.

Diet Colas.
Contain sucralose and acesulfame potassium.

Frozen Dinners.
Contain maltodextrin.

Nonfat Greek Yogurt.
Contains sucralose and acesulfame potassium.

Let's talk about dairy for a second. I do love dairy, but only when it's *clean* dairy. Most dairy products are filled with so many chemicals and hormones.

I just don't feel good when I eat it. Most of the time, I don't eat much dairy at all and that's hard since I love ranch dressing! If you're drinking milk, go for raw dairy from a cow. On the topic of raw milk, I know that certain states have made it illegal, which I think is ridiculous. Virginia, Maryland, New Jersey, West Virginia, North Carolina, Ohio, and Tennessee are just a few. I'm not telling you to do anything illegal, but if you can't drink raw milk it might not be a good idea to have it at all. Use homemade almond or cashew milk for coffee. It's not hard; I recommend using a 2:1 ratio of water to nuts to make sure it's thick enough. Again, there's nothing wrong with dairy if your body can process it. My body struggles with it, but if there's a day that I really want a bowl of nachos, I'll have it.

Crutch Foods

For people who are beginning intermittent fasting for the first time, cutting out all chemicals and artificial sweeteners can be a challenge. Drinking only water, unsweetened tea and black coffee during your fast may even seem impossible at first.

If cutting out all the things you're used to is a major hang-up that's keeping you from starting this plan, then you might need to start with **Crutch Foods**. Crutch Foods are foods that I normally don't recommend you consume while you fast. These foods are only allowed as a starting point until you can progress to a point that you can commit to the fast completely.

Crutch Food Examples

- Bone Broth: If you're going to have bone broth, make sure it's homemade. Those bone broth bouillons are Chemical City.
- Coconut Oil or Heavy Cream in Coffee
- Diet Sodas
- Sugarless Gum/Breath Mints
- Fruit-Flavored Sparkling Water

Remember, this is just a starting point. These kinds of foods will spike your insulin and counteract the purpose of the fast, so you don't want to remain here.

> ### Exodus 15:22-24 (NIV)
> [22] *Then Moses led Israel from the Red Sea and they went into the Desert of Shur. For three days they traveled in the desert without finding water.* [23]*When they came to Marah, they could not drink its water because it was bitter. (That is why the place is called Marah.)* [24] *So the people grumbled against Moses, saying, "What are we to drink?"*

I thought of this verse because of a friend of mine who was trying to stop using Splenda and sugar in her tea. She kept complaining about how bitter tea was without sweetener and I told her she reminded me of this scripture. Over time, her body got used to it and now she drinks unsweetened tea all the time. It was the same for me. I didn't think I could drink unsweetened tea because I found it so disgusting at first. In the beginning, you will grumble a little bit, but keep the Israelites in mind. It's funny because they were only three days into their freedom from Egyptian slavery and already they were complaining! This is going to happen to you when you start fasting. You'll want to grumble and complain, but that's where faith has to kick in.

Principle 8:
Quote God's Word When You Want to Eat, but You're Not Hungry

Matthew 4:4 (NIV)
⁴ Jesus answered, "It is written: 'Man shall not live on bread alone, but on every word that comes from the mouth of God.'"

Feasting on God's Word

You're going to experience great challenges as you desire to eat while you're fasting. You have to know how to fight temptations when they come. We're going to talk about fighting temptation in detail later in this section, but first I want you to understand just how important God's Word is to the success of your fast.

Psalm 119:103 (NIV)

*[103] How sweet are your words to my taste,
sweeter than honey to my mouth!*

I particularly love this verse because, if you haven't noticed by now, I love sweets! I want you to take this verse and substitute honey for whatever your weakness is. Is it cake? Brownies? Pizza? Whatever it is that tempts you, use this scripture to declare your love for God's Word over that food.

"God, I love your words! They are sweeter than ice cream to my mouth! Sweeter than chocolate cake! Sweeter than bread!"

Substitute the Word of God in place of the food. Suddenly, this verse takes on a new meaning because you're feasting on God's Word. Speaking His word is the best tasting treat you could ever have.

You have to change your mindset because most people don't say "MMMMMMM, you know what I would love to have right now? A big dose of Psalms! I am really craving a big taste of Proverbs right now. I think I'm going to stop this car and read the book of Matthew right this second. I want it so bad that I can't even stand it!" Right?

We want to get to the point that we understand that running to food for the answer makes things worse. Turning to anything besides God to fill a void is the wrong answer. Human beings fill their voids with all kinds of vices: gambling, drinking, drugs, illicit sex, and more. As a society, we've been slow to realize that we're doing the same thing with food today. You have to break the cycle. Develop a hunger for the Word like a baby has for breast milk. When my son was a baby, he would go absolutely crazy if he couldn't get to my milk!

Say to yourself, "I know right now that I am not physically hungry. I want to eat for reasons other than nutrition and those are the wrong reasons."

> **Psalm 119:2 (NIV)**
> *2 Blessed are those who keep his statutes
> and seek him with all their heart—*

> **Psalm 119:105 (MSG)**
> *105-112 By your words I can see where I'm going;
> they throw a beam of light on my dark path.*

> **Psalm 119:25 (NIV)**
> *25 I am laid low in the dust;
> preserve my life according to your word.*

The Word of God is the answer when you need to find your way. It's the answer when you're weary and stressed out. There are blessings that come from seeking out the Word instead of other idols. There are so many things that God's Word does for you and it's truly the only thing you need.

You need to speak scriptures during your fast. Here are a few to get you started:

> **Proverbs 23:20-21 (NIV)**
> *20 Do not join those who drink too much wine or gorge
> themselves on meat, 21 for drunkards and gluttons
> become poor, and drowsiness clothes them in rags.*

> **2 Timothy 1:7 (NIV)**
> *7 For the Spirit God gave us does not make us timid,
> but gives us power, love and self-discipline.*

Personalize these scriptures by inserting "I" and "me," where applicable. Ask God to help you adapt the right character traits and dump the bad ones. I have a prayer that you can use as a template to overcome your challenges. Personalize it to fit you:

"God open my eyes and my ears to hear when my stomach is growling. I only want to eat the amount of food today that I require to live. I want to learn how to eat to live, not live to eat. Help me to be sensitive to that exact amount of food so I'm not eating beyond it. Help me take my focus off of food so that I'm not thinking about food constantly. Fill my thoughts with love, joy, and peace instead of fast food and burgers. I'm going to come to you when I'm sad, depressed, anxious or upset. I'm only going to come to you and spend time in Your Word instead of running to brownies."

We All Get Tempted

The fact is, every one of us struggles with temptation. You'll never be so great a person that you stop struggling with it. So, that means you shouldn't be surprised or shocked when temptation comes. Instead be prepared.

**When temptation comes we usually react
with frustration and discouragement.**

"Why do I keep falling in this same area?"

"Why isn't this getting easier?"

"I'll never change!"

"I'm always going to struggle with food!"

You have to stop beating yourself up for being tempted. Being tempted is not a sin! Sin is when you *give in* to the temptation. Even Jesus was tempted, He never sinned. You can't stop the Devil from bombarding your mind with ideas, but you can decide to speak to and get rid of those thoughts.

Have hope! You can get to the place that you're no longer tempted in the area of food. Years ago, I was a smoker. When I was 22 years old, I met a pastor, Vince Antonucci, who invited me to his church, Forefront Church. I told him that I smoked and I wasn't going to give it up. I asked him if he was okay with that and he told me he was. I quit not long after that! Now, there's nothing you can do to get me to smoke. It wasn't that way at first, but now nicotine is not a temptation for me anymore. The same goes for overeating. You can get to the point that you don't like the way overeating feels. Believe that, one day, it won't be a struggle for you anymore.

When you gave your life to Christ you became a target for the Devil. Satan put out a contract on you and has been after you ever since. He wants to see how he can get you to slip, misstep, or fail! Right now, food is a weakness for me, but I'm confident that one day this won't be an area of temptation for me.

In Matthew 26:41a NIV, Jesus said, **"Watch and pray so that you will not fall into temptation."**

So, be prepared! Be watching for it. Be ready for it. Don't be surprised. Know where it's coming from: the Devil! When God gives you an idea in your mind, we call it inspiration or revelation. When the devil gives you an idea in your mind, we call it **temptation**. You get to decide! Which one are you going to be about?

Fighting Temptations

You're going to be tempted to make excuses why it's okay to eat when you're fasting.

"It's my son's birthday."

"I have a group breakfast to go to."

"The family is going out to dinner tonight."

Don't fall for it! Cry out to God instead:

"God, what I want to do right now is eat this entire pan of brownies. But I'm coming to you because I know that I'm not truly hungry right now and it's not my window to eat."

> ## Psalm 81:8-10 (NIV)
> [8] *Hear me, my people, and I will warn you—*
> *if you would only listen to me, Israel!*
> [9] *You shall have no foreign god among you;*
> *you shall not worship any god other than me.*
> [10] *I am the Lord your God,*
> *who brought you up out of Egypt.*
> *Open wide your mouth and I will fill it.*

I know for a fact that temptation comes on strongest when I'm tired. Not getting enough sleep becomes an excuse for me to eat more the next day. We have to be careful about these things because when it comes to temptation:

1. It comes when you least expect it.
2. It comes when you're vulnerable.
3. It comes when you're not spending time with God.

123

Let's use a comparison to show ways that you can resist temptation. Let's compare proper eating with faithfulness in marriage. One thing that I know I would never do is cheat on my husband. There are a few things that I do to ensure that I won't ever do this. These same practices can be applied to your diet.

James 1:14-15 (NIV)
14 but each person is tempted when they are dragged away by their own evil desire and enticed. 15 Then, after desire has conceived, it gives birth to sin...

Proverbs 14:16 (NASB)
16 A wise man...turns away from evil, But a fool is arrogant and careless.

Psalm 119:59-60 (NIV)
59 I have considered my ways and have turned my steps to your statutes. 60 I will hasten and not delay to obey your commands.

Don't get cocky. When you first begin intermittent fasting you might say "I got this! I'll never go back to eating all the time!" Be careful of getting cocky. One of the seasons when we're most vulnerable is after we've had a lot of success. That's when Satan comes in and tempts you big time. Jesus' three temptations by the devil came right after His baptism, a huge success where God came down to support Him publicly. Be alert when things are going really good.

Never blame other people. You need to accept responsibility for your actions and not blame other people. If you cave in and eat too many brownies, admit that it's your own fault. I believe our society lives with a victim mentality. We blame everything and everyone but ourselves for our faults and failures. I can admit that most of my problems were self-inflicted. That's true for me and it's true for you, too.

124

Pray immediately. As soon as you feel tempted, seek God's help in prayer. Don't ponder it. God has a 24-hour hotline system. You can call Him anytime! Some of the greatest prayers for help often look like this:

"God, it's me again. This is the fourth time today I'm coming to you. I had a bad day and I want to go and eat everything in the refrigerator right now, but I know that I can't. Help me to have self-control."

Why does God want you to come to Him? Because He wants you to depend on Him.

> ### Hebrews 4:15-16 (NIV)
> *[15] For we do not have a high priest who is unable to empathize with our weaknesses, but we have one who has been tempted in every way, just as we are—yet he did not sin. [16] Let us then approach God's throne of grace with confidence, so that we may receive mercy and find grace to help us in our time of need.*

We can come boldly without any hesitation or embarrassment because Jesus sympathizes with us. He knows what we're going through. Jesus had the same temptations you do, so you can go to Him with confidence that He can help. Some of you reading this might think this is weird. Maybe it doesn't make sense to you, but it's true. This is what you have to do to succeed at this.

Maybe you think the thing you're missing is more willpower, but willpower only goes so far. It works for a while, but it doesn't last forever. It's not the permanent solution. You can do anything for a little while, but diets can only last for a little while before your willpower fails. You want this to be autopilot. You want it to be your natural tendency to only eat when you're hungry and never eat beyond fullness. Your goal should be to get your body out of willpower mode and into autopilot mode. Get to a place where you aren't thinking hard about every little thing you eat.

When you're face-to-face with your favorite dessert, you're going to call "9-1-1" immediately. You're going to say, "Lord, come help me!"

Surround yourself with accountability partners. You don't have to stand up at work and yell out, "Hey everyone I'm struggling!" but you do need someone you trust. You need someone who will love you, accept you, and pray for you without bringing you down.

If you don't have someone, we can be that for you: Coach@chantelrayway.com

Anybody who is anybody has a coach! Think of your favorite tennis player. Think of you favorite golf pro. They all have coaches to help them get to the next level! Don't lie to yourself and say you don't need help and that you don't really have a problem with food. The fact that you're afraid to admit your weakness in this area is what prevents you from going to the next level. Why do you think people don't want to share their problems with others? It's pride. Pride makes you insecure.

Those secret sins in your life that you're embarrassed about aren't exclusive to you. I promise you, someone else is facing those exact same problems! In fact, God wants us to help each other with these problems. He even made sharing our faults with another person a prerequisite to healing:

James 5:16 (GW)
[16] *So admit your sins to each other...so that you will be healed.*

This isn't something you need to hold in. Tell somebody about it and gain control. Talking about your problem with someone you trust provides support and accountability. You need both of these to be healed of your overeating.

Avoid tempting areas. Stay away from places and scenarios that cause you to stumble. It's common sense that if you don't want to get stung, you stay away from the wasp's nest!

Proverbs 14:16 (NASB)
[16] *A wise man is cautious and turns away from evil, But a fool is arrogant and careless.*

Ephesians 4:27 (NIV)
[27] *and do not give the devil a foothold.*

A fool thinks she can handle everything on her own. Don't be a fool. Recognize your patterns. Where are you most tempted? Is it a certain time of day? Is it on vacation? Business trips? Do you struggle when you're home alone and the kids are gone? Be aware and prepare for these traps.

The Bible instructs us to flee - run away - from temptation. Physically remove yourself from the scene if you have to! Be like Joseph who, in Genesis 39, left his coat and split when Potiphar's wife came onto him. He said, "Sayonara, sucka!" and took off. Be like Joseph, and don't be a fool.

1 Corinthians 10:13 (NIV)
[13] *...And God...will not let you be tempted beyond what you can bear. But when you are tempted, he will also provide a way out so that you can endure it.*

127

"I can't help myself."
"I have to have a late night snack."
"I have to have something early in the morning."

You're calling God a liar every time you say "I can't."
He promises that He'll always provide a way out.

Memorize GOD'S WORD. This is your secret weapon right here. Without a doubt, the #1 single most effective method to combat temptation is to memorize Scripture. This is something that you CAN do. My son is six years old and he has about 150 Bible verses memorized. That's because he recites them every single night. Write scriptures down on little cards or stick them to your mirror. Make yourself a program of memorization. If you have kids, have them memorize them with you.

This is going to be important when you have the Devil in front of you attacking with temptation. If you have no Scripture to fight back with, it's like having a gun with no bullets. When Jesus was tempted in Matthew 3, what did He do? He quoted Scripture! He was showing us how to resist the Devil.

Set up a goal to learn one or two verses a week. If you can't do that, your priorities are messed up. You don't have a time problem; you have a priority problem. Most days I feel like there is not a spare minute in my life, but I still have time to memorize God's Word.

> ### Ephesians 6:17 (NIV)
> *17 Take the helmet of salvation*
> *and the sword of the Spirit,*
> *which is the word of God.*

You are on the battlefield here! You've got to have on the proper armor and you've got to fight for this! This isn't going to be easy.

If you haven't received salvation, you can't use the Word of God as a weapon in this battle. The first step you need to take is to move over and let God be the pilot in your life. Take the co-pilot's seat and accept salvation as your helmet. What does a helmet do? **It protects your mind.** Your weapon in this fight is "the Sword" - those scriptures you memorize from the Word of God.

Say, "Jesus Christ, come into my life. I want to move over and I want you to be the pilot. Give me Your power to use instead of my own. I believe you died on the cross and I want to accept you as Lord of my life. I want to accept responsibility for the temptations that I've been giving in_to in my life. I want to stop making excuses and stop blaming other people. I ask you to help me not eat when I'm not hungry. I want to accept Your salvation today. I want to put on the helmet that will protect my mind. Jesus, I want You to come into my heart and into my life to save me. Forgive me and help me start a brand new life. In Your name, I pray, Amen."

Scriptures to Know

Ephesians 6:17 (NIV)
17 Take the helmet of salvation and the sword of the Spirit, which is the word of God.

1 Corinthians 10:13 (NIV)
13 No temptation has overtaken you except what is common to mankind. And God is faithful; he will not let you be tempted beyond what you can bear. But when you are tempted, he will also provide a way out so that you can endure it.

James 5:16 (GW)
16 So admit your sins to each other...so that you will be healed.

Matthew 26:41a (NIV)
41 "Watch and pray so that you will not fall into temptation.

1 Corinthians 10:12 (NIV)
12 So, if you think you are standing firm, be careful that you don't fall!

Psalm 50:15a (NIV)
15 and call on me in the day of trouble...

4 Steps to Flee Temptation

Step 1 – Flee the scene of temptation immediately.

My routine used to be that I would come home from school or work and have a snack. Now, I stay away from the kitchen when I get home, and I go do something else. If you're at a party with tempting food, don't stand next to the food table. Get yourself away from the scene of temptation.

Step 2 - Remind yourself of your goal.

Keep your eyes on the prize. Tell yourself that you're not eating until your stomach growls.

Step 3 - Immediately pray and quote Bible verses.

Use the scriptures in this section and in the back of this book and start reading out loud. Jesus said that we live by the Word of God and not just bread (Matthew 4:4). Never depend on eating for joy and satisfaction.

Step 4 - Find something else to do.

Start getting your mind off of your own desires. Ask yourself if you're actually hungry. Check to see if your stomach has even growled. Describe your symptoms of hunger and see if you're in the right spot on the hunger scale. True hunger is going to come approximately 1 to 2 times a day depending on how much you eat. You need to change your mindset and delight in being hungry.

> **Psalm 119:103 (NKJV)**
> *103 How sweet are Your words to my taste, Sweeter than honey to my mouth!*

131

It's Sort of Like Marriage

If you're married, there should be certain rules and boundaries that you and your spouse have in place to guard against infidelity. Those same rules apply to how you eat.

1) Set healthy boundaries

I don't go out to eat with or drive in the same car alone with another man. To prevent problems with eating, I create time limits.

2) Avoid vulnerable situations

I don't flirt or have intimate talks with other men. To avoid vulnerability with food, I make sure that I get my sleep and remove the different "stressors" in my life that can cause a problem. And I stay far away from BUFFETS! I just do not do buffets. They are way too overwhelming.

3) Flee the scene

Believe it or not, sometimes I get Facebook messages from strange men.

"OMG, you are drop dead gorgeous!"

"I would love to get to know you!"

Can you guess how I respond? That's right, **DELETE** and **BLOCK!** Right away! It's the same thing with food. If I feel like eating outside of my eating window, I flee the kitchen. I go to my bedroom because that's one of the places I just do not eat. Have safe havens like that in your own home.

132

God Likes to Help

My mom had a saying: "Once the fire gets out of the trash can, you can't put it out!" If you have a small fire in a trash can, you can just dump water on it and it's out. If it's all over the house, then it's like a snowball, moving from room to room. My family had a fire when I was younger that burned down the entire house. It wasn't until the firemen showed up that we discovered it all started from one little spot in the garage.

It's like saying, "I'm just going to kiss this guy" and the next thing you know you're naked! You can't quote scripture at this point. The fire's already gotten all over the house and you can't put it out. Often, we'll make one bad decision with our food and decide to keep eating badly the whole day. "I'll start again tomorrow," becomes the mantra and the snowball keeps growing. That's why it's important to seek God's help before you make the mess.

One time, I was struggling with sticking to my fast and I asked God for help. I was having a Bible study and one of the girls brought vegan cupcakes. I knew these things were delicious and I really wanted one, but I was still in my fast. Suddenly, I smelled smoke. I didn't know where it was coming from at first, but I called 9-1-1. The fire department came and guess where it came from? The garage! Thankfully, nothing burned, but after all of that drama I didn't want the cupcake anymore! We did have to pay for a new hot water heater, but I didn't eat the cupcake! Priorities, right?

I had a similar incident this past weekend at a Cubs reunion party at my home. In this case, I wasn't in the middle of my fast but I was being tempted with some Chemical City cupcakes. If it was a cake made with real ingredients like fresh fruit and real sugar, I would have been happy to eat two or three bites of that. But these cupcakes were just artificial and *blech!*

133

At this party, there were about 20 kids in my dining room. In the dining room were these pretty linen chairs. Right after I prayed for God's help, I looked over and saw blue icing all over my beautiful linen. The sight of that took my mind right off of eating cupcakes! I was consumed with cleaning now.

Distractions are great! I can put ice cream that I know I don't need to be eating in a bowl and my son will call my name before I can take my first bite. That happened once before and when I got back the ice cream was melted to mush and I didn't want it anymore.

God uses lots of distractions and even mishaps with me. I was recently at a meal with friends during my fast. I justified my desire to eat by extending my eating window to eight hours even though I had committed to six. I ordered chicken tacos, but the restaurant mixed up my order and brought me fish tacos instead. I can't stand fish! The waitress offered to bring me the right food, but I refused. I saved money and I didn't violate my fast!

If you earnestly pray in the morning, "God protect me from myself, and make it so I don't eat these kinds of things" He will help you. I was going to disobey, but He made it so I would obey. Instead of getting frustrated, I chuckled.

I love being a Christian because God has a sense of humor, and helps us with the little things in life. A lot of people think God is only concerned with big things, but that's not true! He wants to be a part of every little thing in your life including what you eat. This kind of relationship with God strengthens us as we learn to trust Him more and more. Involving him in what you eat is like inviting Him to your every meal!

Escape Routes

Don't eat your first meal until your stomach growls. When you're tempted to eat, pray for your way of escape.

> ## 1 Corinthians 10:13 (NIV)
> *[13] No temptation has overtaken you except what is common to mankind. And God is faithful; he will not let you be tempted beyond what you can bear. But when you are tempted, he will also provide a way out so that you can endure it.*

When I'm not hungry but I want to eat, I cry out to God, "where is my escape route?" God will provide that way out.

One time, I prayed for an escape route from my daughter's birthday cake. The cake was really good and the leftovers were sitting in the kitchen on the countertop. I was tempted to eat some and I really needed an escape! While cleaning up, I tried to push it out of my way and half of it fell in the sink! It was an accident, but it was exactly what I needed. I didn't want it anymore after that!

It happened again with my favorite brand of chips. I was eating way too many straight from the bag when my son came by and tried to snatch some. The bag tore apart and they spilled out all over the floor. If my son didn't snatch them when he did, I might have eaten the whole bag.

We need to remember that food is not for comfort and it's not a reward. There's a saying that goes, "nothing tastes as good as skinny feels" and, in a sense, that's true. One hour of indulging myself is not going to end well for me. So, I created the habit of not eating until my stomach growls with my first meal and I ask God for my escape route.

Genesis 9:3 (NIV)
3 Everything that lives and moves about will be food for you. Just as I gave you the green plants, I now give you everything.

All Food is Acceptable

There are many scriptures in the Bible that make it clear that all foods are acceptable to eat. In my mind, that means any real foods (not chemicals) are free to eat and shouldn't be altogether restricted from any person's diet.

1 Timothy 4:1-5 (NASB)
4 But the Spirit explicitly says that in later times some will fall away from the faith, paying attention to deceitful spirits and doctrines of demons, 2 by means of the hypocrisy of liars seared in their own conscience as with a branding iron, 3 men who forbid marriage and advocate abstaining from foods which God has created to be gratefully shared in by those who believe and know the truth. 4 For everything created by God is good, and nothing is to be rejected if it is received with gratitude; 5 for it is sanctified by means of the word of God and prayer.

Now, I don't go so far as saying that every one who promotes a diet is demonic, but I do believe that it's wrong for anyone to call it a sin to eat a particular food. My goal with this book is to free you from being too focused on food and to help you stop being a diet-chaser.

We all have personal convictions on how we should eat. For me, it's very important to eat real foods with no chemicals. On top of that, there are certain foods like dairy and gluten I eat in limited amounts because they have a negative affect on my health. However, I would never call my eating habits a law that everyone else must follow. You can eat however you're led to eat. Some people may feel the need to eat vegan or vegetarian, but no one can require that of another person. The only restriction God places on food is concerning the amount that you eat.

Deuteronomy 12:15, 20, 21, 26 (NASB)

[15]*"However, you may slaughter and eat meat within any of your gates, whatever you desire, according to the blessing of the Lord your God which He has given you; the unclean and the clean may eat of it, as of the gazelle and the deer.*

[20] *"When the Lord your God extends your border as He has promised you, and you say, 'I will eat meat,' because you desire to eat meat, then you may eat meat, whatever you desire.*

[21] *If the place which the Lord your God chooses to put His name is too far from you, then you may slaughter of your herd and flock which the Lord has given you, as I have commanded you; and you may eat within your gates whatever you desire.*
[26] *Only your holy things which you may have and your votive offerings, you shall take and go to the place which the Lord chooses.*

Mark 7:18-20 (NASB)

[18] *And He *said to them, "Are you so lacking in understanding also? Do you not understand that whatever goes into the man from outside cannot defile him,* [19] *because it does not go into his heart, but into his stomach, and is eliminated?" (Thus He declared all foods clean.)* [20] *And He was saying, "That which proceeds out of the man, that is what defiles the man.*

137

Deciding How to Eat

Among Christians, there are many different opinions on veganism and vegetarianism. Some of them can be extreme. I have a friend that we'll call "Corey." Corey is so passionate about not eating meat that she believes anyone who does is a sinner. There can be a lot of emotion surrounding this topic, but intolerance for the different ways people eat bothers me.

I feel there is scriptural support for people who want to eat a vegan, vegetarian, or meat-inclusive diet. You have to pray and get wisdom from the Bible and find out what God wants you to do. The New Testament makes it very clear that every individual needs to follow his or her own conscience when it comes to eating. Make your own decision even if others disagree.

Genesis 1:29-30 (NIV)
29 Then God said, "I give you every seed-bearing plant on the face of the whole earth and every tree that has fruit with seed in it. They will be yours for food. 30 And to all the beasts of the earth and all the birds in the sky and all the creatures that move along the ground—everything that has the breath of life in it—I give every green plant for food." And it was so.

Many Christians who are vegan or vegetarian believe that this passage is God's original plan and purpose for how we ought to eat. They model their eating habits after these scriptures.

Genesis 9:3 (NIV)
3 Everything that lives and moves about will be food for you. Just as I gave you the green plants, I now give you everything.

Leviticus 11:2-3 (NIV)
...Of all the animals that live on land, these are the ones you may eat: 3 You may eat any animal that has a divided hoof and that chews the cud.

On the other hand, the following passages clearly allow for the consumption of meat as well as reveal foods God wants you to avoid.

Mark 7:18-19 (NIV)
[18] "Are you so dull?" he asked. "Don't you see that nothing that enters a person from the outside can defile them? [19] For it doesn't go into their heart but into their stomach, and then out of the body." (In saying this, Jesus declared all foods clean.)

Finally, we see Jesus doing away with all of the previous rules about food. God delivered a similar message to Peter in the Book of Acts while he was on the rooftop of Simon the Tanner's house in Joppa (Acts 10).

Peter was told...

Acts 10:15 (NIV)
"...Do not call anything impure that God has made clean."

The Bible also addresses how we should treat each other in regard to the foods we eat:

> ## Romans 14:2-3, 6 (NIV)
> *2 One person's faith allows them to eat anything, but another, whose faith is weak, eats only vegetables. 3The one who eats everything must not treat with contempt the one who does not, and the one who does not eat everything must not judge the one who does, for God has accepted them. 6 Whoever eats meat does so to the Lord, for they give thanks to God; and whoever abstains does so to the Lord and gives thanks to God.*

It's worth mentioning that some Christians recommend a vegetarian diet not because of Scripture, but because of the treatment of animals in the food industry. This is a point worth considering. God gave us dominion over all the earth (Genesis 1:28), but He also expects us to behave responsibly and be accountable for the way we treat His creation.

> ## Proverbs 12:10a (NIV)
> *10 The righteous care for the needs of their animals*

I think animal rights groups have a very valid point in that we need to treat animals with respect, but, unfortunately, many of them have forgotten that animal life cannot be given priority over human life. I know some people who would rather starve to death than eat animal meat. If that's you, I respect that! You should also respect those who choose to eat meat.

Below are a series of scriptures to consider while you're deciding how you want to eat and how to handle people who eat differently from you.

> ## Isaiah 25:6 (NIV)
> *6 On this mountain the Lord Almighty will prepare a feast of rich food for all peoples, a banquet of aged wine— the best of meats and the finest of wines.*

140

Genesis 1:30 (NRSV)

30 And to every beast of the earth, and to every bird of the air, and to everything that creeps on the earth, everything that has the breath of life, I have given every green plant for food." And it was so.

Daniel 1:8, 11-12, 15 (NIV)

But Daniel resolved not to defile himself with the royal food and wine...
Daniel then said..."Give us nothing but vegetables to eat and water to drink...At the end of the ten days they looked healthier and better nourished than any of the young men who ate the royal food.

Isaiah 65:25 (NRSV)

25 The wolf and the lamb shall feed together, the lion shall eat straw like the ox; but the serpent—its food shall be dust! They shall not hurt or destroy on all my holy mountain, says the LORD.

Job 12:7 (NRSV)

7 "But ask the animals, and they will teach you; the birds of the air, and they will tell you;

Proverbs 12:10 (NRSV)

10 The righteous know the needs of their animals, but the mercy of the wicked is cruel.

Psalm 147:9 (NRSV)

*⁹ He gives to the animals their food, and
to the young ravens when they cry.*

Hosea 2:18 (NRSV)

*¹⁸ I will make for you a covenant on that day with the wild
animals, the birds of the air, and the creeping things of
the ground; and I will abolish the bow, the sword, and
war from the land; and I will make you lie down in safety.*

Jeremiah 12:4 (NRSV)

*⁴ How long will the land mourn,
and the grass of every field wither?
or the wickedness of those who live in it
the animals and the birds are swept away,
and because people said,
"He is blind to our ways."*

Luke 12:6 (NRSV)

*⁶ Are not five sparrows sold for two pennies?
Yet not one of them is forgotten in God's sight.*

Psalm 36:6 (NRSV)

*⁶ Your righteousness is like the mighty mountains,
your judgments are like the great deep; you save
humans and animals alike, O LORD.*

Matthew 5:7 (NRSV)

*⁷ "Blessed are the merciful, for
they will receive mercy.*

Pros and Cons of Vegan and Vegetarian Diets

I feel my best when I eat tons of fruits and vegetables. There are vitamins, fiber, and vital nutrients that only come from plant sources. Simply put, the more vegetables you eat the healthier you're going to be!

A **vegetarian** diet tends to be lower in calories and fat. Most of the fats encountered in the vegetarian diet are the "good" kind. To be specific, they are **monounsaturated fats**. In practical terms, this means that they lower LDL (the "bad" cholesterol) and may raise HDL ("good" cholesterol).

On the other hand, strict vegetarians and vegans may fail to get enough protein and essential amino acids in their diets. If you're going to be on a vegetarian or vegan diet, you should definitely consult a registered dietitian or your doctor to make sure you're getting all the nutrients your body needs.

What Works for Your Body

At this point, it's clear that the Bible says there aren't any foods you're lawfully restricted from eating. In fact, in Genesis 18, God sat down with Abraham and ate red meat, butter and raw milk! However, that doesn't mean you should still eat any and everything. Because even though you're *allowed* to eat anything, your body may not *agree* with everything.

You have to find out what you can and can't eat for your body specifically. The Bible says I can eat bread and milk, but I don't eat a lot of it because my body doesn't process gluten and dairy very well. I just eat it in limited amounts and I feel fine.

143

The Paleo Diet

I want to take a moment to discuss the **paleo diet**. Like veganism or vegetarianism, I absolutely don't think eating this way should be a requirement for anyone. However, I would highly recommend a version of paleo for anyone suffering from an autoimmune disease like me. I have Hashimoto's disease, an autoimmune disease that attacks the thyroid. Whenever I ate 100% paleo, my condition got drastically better. Now, I do an 80/20 style of paleo combined with my intermittent fasting. This combination has actually cured my condition and I no longer take any medication for my thyroid.

A quick note: if you research the paleo diet, you'll find arguments that it is an evolutionary diet based on cavemen and so Christians should not eat that way. I don't see paleo as a religion. Christian is what I am and paleo is simply what I eat and nothing more.

The Paleo-ish Method

The modern American diet isn't very good. It's full of chemicals and foods that lead us to autoimmune diseases, thyroid problems, cancer, digestive disorders, and heart disease. How and what you eat affects your health, and my personal health problems are what led me to eat what I call **paleo-ish**.

NOTE: This section is for people who suffer from an autoimmune disease and would like to know what I did to cure my condition. If you don't suffer from any of these problems, then you have no reason to eat paleo-ish. The 80/20 rule is just fine for you. As always, talk to your doctor before making any decisions.

Paleo-ish is simply paleo with a few personal differences. The paleo diet basically tells you to eat lean meat and fruits and vegetables that even the Bible tells you to eat. Very simply, paleo is clean eating.

Now, there are three different ways I think you can do this:

Pure Paleo

No grains, dairy, soy or refined or processed foods.

80/20 Paleo

80% of the time you're eating paleo.
20% of the time you're eating whatever you want.

Auto-Immune Paleo

For people with chronic autoimmune disorders like fibromyalgia, psoriasis, lupus, IBS and more, there are certain foods in the paleo diet that can't be eaten. Depending on your health issue, you will have to test out different foods and find out what you respond well to.

Before I came across paleo, I was overweight with dry skin, debilitating fatigue, and brittle hair that was falling out. My doctor told me that I had autoimmune hypothyroidism caused by Hashimoto's Thyroiditis. Paleo is how I healed that.

I started out doing paleo 100% without even knowing how much effect it would have on my thyroid. I actually felt terrible at first because my thyroid kicked into overdrive and reacted to my medication. I could physically tell that I needed to back off of my medication. I lowered it and stopped doing paleo 100%. That sent me on a roller coaster for a while until I found my balance of an 80/20 paleo diet or paleo-ish.

I began at 125mg of Synthroid medication for my thyroid, but I was able to bring that down incrementally until I didn't have to take it at all. My doctor was surprised that my eating was the only change that I made. My psoriasis even got better. This all happened because of eating paleo-ish combined with intermittent fasting. The two worked together and I wouldn't have gotten these results without both of them.

Foods allowed on paleo:

Meats of any kind
grass fed or pasture raised

Seafood
wild caught

Vegetables
organic and local

Eggs

Fruit
organic

Nuts and seeds of all kinds
in moderation

Fat
preferably avocado oils, coconut oils, extra virgin olive oil, and ghee

Paleo-friendly sweeteners
raw honey, maple syrup, coconut sugar, coconut nectar, and dates

Foods to limit:

Grains
gluten and non-gluten

Legumes
all beans, soy, and peanuts

Dairy
milk, creamers, cheeses, and yogurts

Processed and Refined Foods

For more information on thyroid health, go to: www.ChantelRayWay.com/thyroid

I want to make a note about dairy. I have friends who choose to eat only raw, unprocessed dairy and that seems to work for them. Personally, I love dairy, but the less I have, the better I do. I can only have dairy here and there as part of my 3 bite rule (we'll discuss that later). If I have any more than that, my body just can't handle it. The one dairy you can have that's part of paleo is ghee. Most people can tolerate it better than butter because it's pure fat.

Once again, none of these restrictions apply to you if your health isn't negatively impacted by any of these foods. You're free to eat whatever you want. Nowhere in the Bible does it say "thou shall not have dairy or gluten!" What the Bible does say is this:

> ### 1 Corinthians 10:23 (NIV)
> [23] *"I have the right to do anything," you say—but not everything is beneficial. "I have the right to do anything"—but not everything is constructive.*

I'm not here to tell you what you can and cannot have. I can tell you what works for me and you have to find out what is beneficial for you.

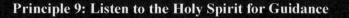

God's Power vs My Power

The excuse many people give for why they can't stick to this plan is a lack of willpower.

"I don't have the willpower to only eat half a candy bar. I can't eat just five M&Ms. I don't have the strength to stop eating and put my food away."

Instead of relying on your self-discipline, you need to rely on *God's* discipline. Many of us were taught to live the Christian life wrong. I was taught about this "Christian wheel" method when I first became a Christian. The idea was that, if you wanted to be a good Christian, there were certain things you had to do. You had to go to church every Sunday, pray, fellowship with other Christians, evangelize, and spend time in the Word of God. If you did those things, then you would have a fruitful Christian life. The part people miss is that you have to live your life through **the power of the Holy Spirit.** You have to do everything with the Lord's help.

True Christian discipline sounds like this, "God, will you please help me get through this? I can't do this without you. I realize I am completely weak in this area. Without You, I can't turn from my old ways. I need Your help to do this."

Living your life with the help of the Holy Spirit is the only way to succeed. While all the things in that wheel are good, they're tools. They're not a substitute for the power of God.

> **Matthew 11:18-19 (NIV)**
> [18] *For John came neither eating nor drinking, and they say, 'He has a demon.' [19] The Son of Man came eating and drinking, and they say, 'Here is a glutton and a drunkard, a friend of tax collectors and sinners.' But wisdom is proved right by her deeds."*

Accountability and Strongholds

In order to overcome gluttony, you have to be honest with yourself. In today's society, we call just about everything a disease. It may not be a popular point of view, but I don't see overeating and alcoholism as diseases. These things are avoidable. If you never have a drink, you can never become an alcoholic. So, it's the same with overeating. There are choices you made that put you in the position you find yourself in now. You have to learn to take personal responsibility for where you are and learn self-control.

Accountability and **self-control** are a huge part of this journey. If you don't stop blaming others for where you are, you're never going to take responsibility for your life and overcome your struggle.

To take control of your actions, you have to start with taking control of your thoughts. The Bible talks about taking thoughts captive in 2 Corinthians 10:5. It's one of the most important things you can do when it comes to weight loss. Your mind is a battlefield. It's where you fight those battles of *should I?* or *shouldn't I?*

I know I shouldn't overeat but that pan of brownies looks really good right now!

149

> ## 2 Corinthians 10:5-6 (NIV)
> *⁵ We demolish arguments and every pretension that sets itself up against the knowledge of God, and we take captive every thought to make it obedient to Christ. ⁶ And we will be ready to punish every act of disobedience, once your obedience is complete.*

A thought left uncaptured eventually becomes a stronghold. We get a picture in our minds of the thing that we want and then we can't seem to get free from it. Biblical fasting is so powerful because it can free you from your strongholds.

Let's look at examples of different strongholds we develop in our lives:

Scenario 1:

Pizza, your favorite food, pops up in your mind. You think about it for a while and now you can't get the image out. Now, all you can think is pizza, pizza, pizza until you finally eat it.

Scenario 2:

You go to a buffet and eat six times what you normally do. You do this because you rationalize that you have to eat your money's worth.

Scenario 3:

You decide you can't fast in the morning because someone told you a long time ago that you have to eat breakfast to have enough energy to survive the day.

Scenario 4:

You don't fast because you have a firm belief that if you ever get hungry, you'll get cranky.

2 Corinthians instructs us to take these thoughts captive and bring them to the Lord. If fasting is mentioned 77 times in the Bible, then I think it's meant to be a major part of our Christian lives. If God told us to do it, then it's something we can do successfully.

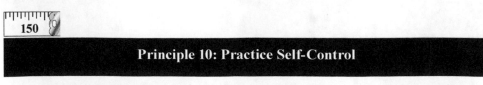

150

Matthew 9:15 (NIV)

15 Jesus answered, "How can the guests of the bridegroom mourn while he is with them? The time will come when the bridegroom will be taken from them; then they will fast.

Acts 13:2 (NIV)

2 While they were worshiping the Lord and fasting, the Holy Spirit said, "Set apart for me Barnabas and Saul for the work to which I have called them."

Acts 14:23 (NIV)

23 Paul and Barnabas appointed elders for them in each church and, with prayer and fasting, committed them to the Lord, in whom they had put their trust.

In the first passage, we see Jesus telling us that his disciples will be people that fast. In the next two, we learn that whenever Jesus' followers fast, it brings clarity. When you're trying to break a stronghold in your life, you need to **pray** and **fast**.

Philippians 4:8 (NIV)

8 Finally, brothers and sisters, whatever is true, whatever is noble, whatever is right, whatever is pure, whatever is lovely, whatever is admirable—if anything is excellent or praiseworthy—think about such things.

Proverbs 12:5 (NIV)

5 The plans of the righteous are just, but the advice of the wicked is deceitful.

151

We have to think positively and overcome negative thoughts. Start with prayer and ask God to bring negative thoughts to your attention, so that you can get rid of them. Pray for a mind that thinks thoughts like Philippians 4:8 and actually quote the scripture. Start your day with a devotional in God's Word to equip yourself to win. In your idle time, when negative thoughts start to creep in, listen to praise and worship music or to our podcast. Cancel those thoughts out immediately when they arise.

God's Rules
vs
Man's Rules

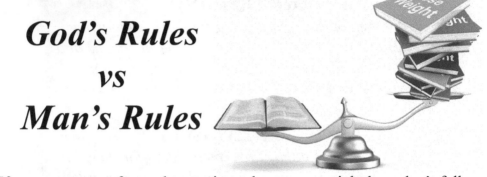

If you ever get unfocused or anxious about your weight loss, don't follow the temptation to try another of the world's man-made quick fix diets. You have to go back to the Biblical principles for eating whenever this happens. If the diet doesn't encourage you to refrain from gluttony, not make food an idol, and operate in balance and self-control then it's not for you.

If you talk to a friend who's doing a low-carb diet and losing a ton of weight overnight, you're going to be tempted to do the same. Diets and restrictions are all man-made rules designed to keep you in bondage. These rules are as subtle as feeling required to eat breakfast just because everyone told you to. If you're not hungry, why eat? Why submit yourself to that bondage? Dieting – the practice of restricting what you can and can't eat – is slavery. It's creating a false god.

We have to focus our minds on God's way for our lives and not man's way. After reading every scripture on food there is over and over again, I discovered that they all fall into the 10 principles you've read in Part II of this book. That's God's way.

Don't let yourself get sidetracked no matter how hard it might be to stay focused. If you lose 3 pounds this week, don't decide that you've "earned" the right to not work as hard next week. That's a textbook trap right there! Pray every day that God will keep you focused.

The Devil is going to tell you different lies, but you can't listen to them. He'll say things like, "You had a rough day, and you deserve to eat."

"You're not feeling well, so you need food to make you feel better."

"You have so much weight to lose that it's hopeless!"

"You're full, but one or two more bites won't hurt."

"Don't wait too long to eat or it'll mess up your metabolism."

When you hear these kinds of things you have to combat them with Scripture.

> ### John 15:5 (NIV)
> [5] *"I am the vine; you are the branches. If you remain in me and I in you, you will bear much fruit; apart from me you can do nothing.*

Combine Scripture with positive statements that combat the negative ones you hear in your mind.

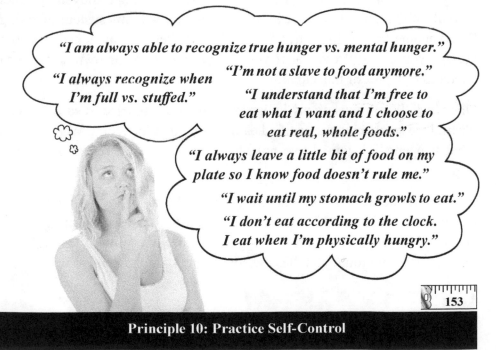

"I am always able to recognize true hunger vs. mental hunger."

"I always recognize when I'm full vs. stuffed."

"I'm not a slave to food anymore."

"I understand that I'm free to eat what I want and I choose to eat real, whole foods."

"I always leave a little bit of food on my plate so I know food doesn't rule me."

"I wait until my stomach growls to eat."

"I don't eat according to the clock. I eat when I'm physically hungry."

153

I want to address a couple of common myths people believe about eating that just aren't true. These are things you need to drop from your thinking.

MYTH: Late night eating will stop you from losing weight.

I have a ton of friends who don't eat anything all day long. They wait until 8:30 at night to eat with their spouses because they get home late. These girls are stick thin!

MYTH: You have to eat every couple of hours.

We're watching people not eat breakfast and go long periods of time without eating and still lose weight. The Bible doesn't say anything about breakfast being the most important meal of the day. Your body knows just how much oxygen it needs to live, and it knows how much food it needs, too. Listen to it!

Galatians 4:9 (NIV)

⁹ But now that you know God—or rather are known by God—how is it that you are turning back to those weak and miserable forces? Do you wish to be enslaved by them all over again?

Tell yourself that there is no alternative. Instead of being enslaved by a diet, take all of that energy and focus on obeying God and his system of eating. Stop running from self-control. Even with the Weight Watchers diet's point system you can still overeat if you're not careful. Your own self-control needs to be a part of this equation.

One week, I lost focus on my hunger and fullness and tried to eat very, very clean. I ate so clean that I justified eating more than I needed. Want to guess what happened? I gained two pounds! I lost focus and fell into a dieting trap.

Dieting produces drastic weight swings. When I was dieting I was constantly gaining and losing 10-15 pounds. You could find sizes 6-10 in my closet because I never knew where I was going to be. Intermittent fasting is the only system I've found that has me consistently losing weight.

154

Mindful Eating

Maintaining your weight loss isn't just about what you eat, it's about why you eat and what you do when you eat it. There are plenty of times that we eat when we aren't actually hungry.

We eat because we're tired, sad, or angry. We're using food to tranquilize our emotions. If you can't admit to that kind of behavior you will never, ever get free from the addiction of food. Emotional eating is a habit we have to break. Your new #1 habit should be to listen to your physical hunger and stop eating when you're full. If you learn these habits, then you'll have what you need to succeed.

I love intermittent fasting because it taught me to be a more mindful eater. The mindful eater asks herself the right questions, and the most important question she asks is, "why am I eating?" We should only eat for physical hunger and not because we're angry, lonely, bored, stressed, anxious, or depressed. Those emotional cues override your internal signal of actual hunger and fullness. Those cues teach you to view food as a comfort.

You don't even know when to stop eating because you weren't hungry when you started! You just keep going until the food is gone. This is a huge deal. The "why am I eating" question is a speed bump that makes you slow down and take a moment to recognize what's going on. It makes you identify the emotional cue that's driving you to eat.

Principle 10: Practice Self-Control

Another important question a mindful eater asks is this:

"Am I physically hungry?"

Learn to recognize the physical signs of true hunger. Is your stomach growling? Does it feel hollow and empty? If not, you need to redirect your attention with one of the following activities:

- **Pray**
- **Play Christian music**
- **Take a shower/bath**
- **Pet your dog**
- **Talk on the phone with a friend**
- **Read God's Word**
- **Brush your teeth**
- **Take a walk**
- **Hug your children**

Once those questions are answered in the right way - you're eating because you're hungry - then ask yourself these questions while you eat:

1. *Am I eating distracted?*

Don't be a distracted eater. Watching TV is an activity that can distract you from listening to your body's signals and you can easily overeat. While you're eating, focus on the food and listen to your body.

2. *Am I fueling my body with real food?*

Stay on track with eating real, whole foods that aren't full of chemicals.

3. *Am I stopping right before I'm full?*

You should never stuff yourself. Ask yourself how you want to feel when you're done eating. Good, energetic and satisfied? Or tired, stuffed and bad like you want to take a nap? I don't want to feel bad, so I don't want to supersize my portions. I want to make sure that I'm eating 30-50% less than what I was eating before.

Enjoying Food Isn't a Sin

As we talk about being disciplined and having self-control, I don't want you to think that food is the enemy. In fact, putting whole groups of food in a "hands off" zone makes you want it more. It's kind of like with Adam and Eve when God said "you can't have this one tree," then all Eve could think about was eating fruit from that one tree. As soon as someone says you can't have it, that's all you think about.

Enjoying food is not a sin. I don't believe your attitude has to be "I can only eat to live and I can't enjoy anything that I eat." I don't agree with that! I think you can enjoy food in moderation. You don't want to have this frantic mentality that obsesses over every detail about food:

"OK, what am I going to have for lunch? I don't want a sandwich (but I do) because it has too many carbs. I don't want to have this croissant with chocolate (but I do) because it has too much sugar. I don't want a frittata (oh, yes I do!) because it has too many eggs and they have cholesterol."

You can just get so crazy about it! I personally think that chocolate is not from the Devil and God hasn't restricted you from eating it. I believe you can have healthy and yummy together. It's just all about portion control. A lot of people pray a general prayer when they sit down to eat.

"Thank You for this food and help it to be nourishing to my body."

Instead, pray with a purpose:

"Thank You for the food You put in front of me. Help me not to feel guilty about eating any of it, but to eat in moderation. Help me to know when my body is full. Help me to stop before I overeat and give me supernatural power to show restraint and self-control."

157

The Holy Spirit should be your personal nutritionist. Invite Him to your meal! By the time you're done with this book, if nothing else, you should be praying much more honestly.

Proverbs 29:18 (NIV)
18 Where there is no revelation, people cast off restraint; but blessed is the one who heeds wisdom's instruction.

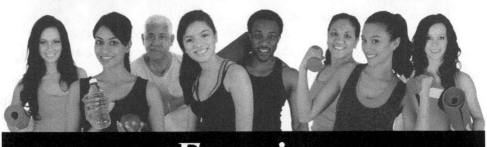

Exercise

1 Timothy 4:8 (NIV)
8 For physical training is of some value

That scripture, in my opinion, means that you should be exercising in some form as long as you are physically able. You should be doing some sort of exercise at least three times a week and I personally think weight training is the way to go. I have lots of friends that don't do any cardio at all but are in great shape and great health. I personally workout every single day because I feel so much better when I do. However, your weight loss is 90% diet and 10% exercise. That's why this book is focused on your eating. My number one goal is to get you eating right!

The one thing I want to warn you about exercise – especially cardio – is to never use it as an excuse to eat more. If your only justification to eat something is that you'll "work it off" later, then don't eat it!

Triggers

My mom is coming into town this week and I was reminded that when I'm with my mom I tend to overeat a little bit. My mom eats *so* healthy. She is one of those people that has two boiled eggs for breakfast, a grilled chicken salad for lunch and salmon and vegetables for dinner. So, I think I try to be healthier when I'm with her and end up not eating enough to be satisfied which leads to overeating. If she gets a grilled chicken salad, I'll get one too even though that's not really what I want. Because it doesn't satisfy me, I snack on dark chocolate and nuts and fruit when I get home. This is a "trigger" for me, so I have to be very aware of it and not fall into that trap. One of my other triggers is when I visit my aunt. My family is from Iran and Iranians have this thing where they want you to EAT, EAT, EAT! You want them to think you like it, so you eat as much as you can.

Types of Triggers

1 ***Behavioral Triggers*** - Behavioral triggers are things you do that make you want to eat. Every night my son and I watch at least two episodes of his favorite show "Good Luck Charlie." Every night, he always says, "Let's get a movie snack." That's an example of a behavioral trigger. In his mind, when it's time to watch the show it's also time to get a snack. So, I have to ask him, "are you really hungry? We just ate dinner a little while ago." I used to have a behavioral trigger when I was younger where right after I got home from school or work I would go straight to the kitchen and get something to eat. Now, I don't go to the kitchen first when I get home. Set up rules and boundaries that will circumvent those behaviors. I can decide that, instead of going to the kitchen, I'm going to go and take a hot bath, first. If you're truly hungry, then eat, but you need to challenge your behaviors and ask yourself what's really going on first.

2 ***Emotional Triggers -*** Emotional triggers can come from a bunch of different sources. My main emotional triggers are anger, bad news at work, feeling down in the dumps, or even just feeling like I deserve food because I worked so hard. An example of a work frustration happened very recently. My web designer for Chantel Ray Real Estate was offered by a different company $40,000 more than what he was making with us. It was so frustrating because we had finally found a great web guy but we couldn't afford to keep him. That was an emotional trigger for me.

3 ***Environmental Triggers -*** An environmental trigger can be anything from seeing a TV commercial of people eating to coworkers bringing in brownies to everyone going out to happy hour. These unexpected scenarios pop up and make you want to be a participant and not feel left out.

> ### 1 Corinthians 10:13 (NIV)
> *¹³ No temptation has overtaken you except what is common to mankind. And God is faithful; he will not let you be tempted beyond what you can bear. But when you are tempted, he will also provide a way out so that you can endure it.*

What you have to do is really pay attention and ask yourself, "what is my trigger?" When the trigger shows up, immediately quote 1 Corinthians 10:13 and make a decision:

"Am I going to run to God, or am I going to run to food? If I run to God, I will gain a lasting satisfaction that truly fulfills me."

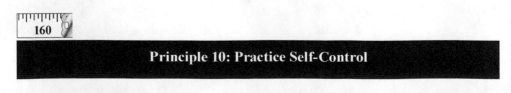

Self-Talk

Positive self-talk is, in my opinion, one of the greatest things you can ever learn how to do. Even when I was heavy, my friends always told me that you'd think I was a runway model just because I carried myself with so much confidence. Anyone can walk in this sort of confidence no matter what they look like. I have a friend who says that when he walks into a room, in his mind, he's 6'3" and 200lbs of pure muscle. He's actually 5'4" and bald! Tell yourself what to think about yourself, and, if you have to, pretend you are better than what you are.

We're all our own toughest critics, but we also lie to ourselves more than we do anyone else. You tell yourself things that are not true and you believe them! Your consciousness influences your identity, so if you're constantly telling yourself things like-

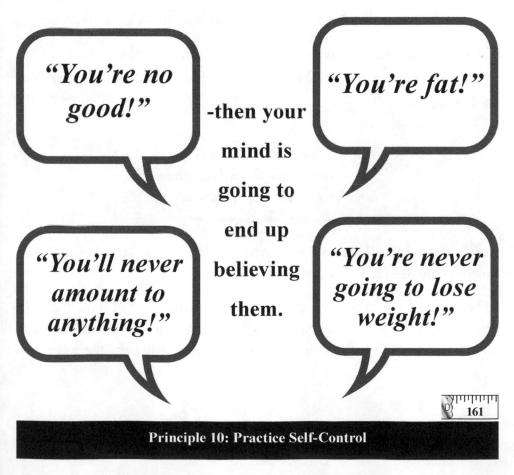

"You're no good!"

-then your mind is going to end up believing them.

"You're fat!"

"You'll never amount to anything!"

"You're never going to lose weight!"

161

> **Proverbs 23:7 (NKJV)**
> [7] *For as he thinks in his heart, so is he...*
> *Whatever you think of yourself is how you will turn out.*

> **Proverbs 4:23 (NCV)**
> [23] *Be careful what you think, because your thoughts run your life.*

If you want to run in a different direction, you have to **change your thoughts**. There's a phrase my husband tells me all the time (probably several times a week). He says, "Just because you feel that way doesn't mean it's true."

If you keep saying negative things to yourself and thinking them in your mind over and over, these fears and thoughts become self-fulfilling. You're sabotaging yourself!

> **Job 3:25 (MSG)**
> [25] *The worst of my fears has come true, what I've dreaded most has happened.*

You have to be really careful with what you're saying. Here is something positive you need to tell yourself:

"The reason I didn't lose weight before is because I didn't have the right plan. Now, I have the right plan, and I'm going to lose weight. Now, I'm committed to eating less food, and the less food that I eat the more I'm going to lose."

Running to God

The reason that people really struggle during their fast is because they aren't running to God during that time. That's the number one problem! You can do the fast all day, but if you're not going to God, it's not going to work.

We want to eat and think like a thin eater. A thin eater doesn't eat diet food. She eats when she's hungry and she stops eating when she's full. You want to eat 30-50% of the amount of food you used to. If you shorten your window but eat the same amount of food as you always did, you won't lose as much weight as you want to. You have to consume less food.

I went to the doctor's office the other day and I saw a very thin lady with a big bowl of candy on her desk. I thought to myself that in most cases having that candy just sitting there would be a huge issue. That's not the case for someone with self-control. She can literally have that candy there and it won't affect her in any way, shape, or form.

I'm not a big alcohol drinker. I probably drink 3 times a year, if that, because I don't like to drink my calories. So, I could have every kind of liquor at my desk and not be tempted to touch it. While that wouldn't be the case for someone else, it just doesn't have a pull on me. That's a sign that you no longer have that magnetic attraction to food when you can have something like a jar of candy on your desk and not even be moved by it.

You want to get to the point that, unless you're hungry, you're not thinking about food. That means you have to turn to God for comfort when that temptation arises.

A diet makes you focus on food *more*. "What am I eating? What's in it? What are the ingredients?"

When you say, "I'm not going to have this," you suddenly start thinking about that particular food over and over again. So, with this plan, you can eat whatever you want. There is nothing you can't have. You're simply learning how to eat "non-clean" foods in moderation. You want your body to talk to you about what you're craving and what you're eating. You want to learn to listen to God's voice instructing you what to eat and what not to eat.

The question you always have to ask yourself is this: "Does my *stomach* need food or do my *emotions* need food?" Here's the truth:

You will never be able to give yourself enough food to satisfy your emotions.

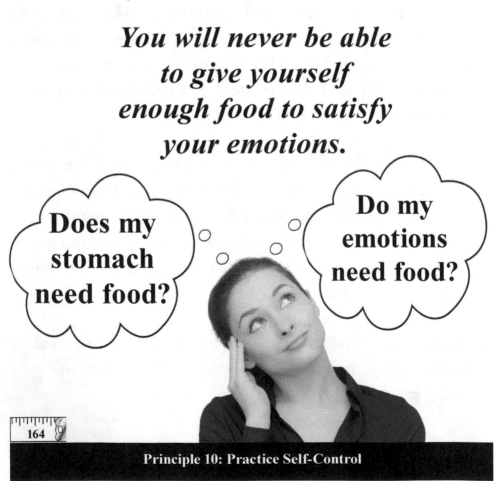

Principle 10: Practice Self-Control

Work Ethic, Image Ethic, and Eating Ethic

There are certain things in life that just come naturally for certain people. Personally, I've always been a hard worker and having a good work ethic is something that's really important to me. That's where I got my "attaboys" from when I was young.

I was employee of the month 6 months in a row at the Burger King I worked at when I was 14. It all happened because I was really good at math. This particular Burger King had two drive-thru windows but they were too cheap to put a register at the second window. So, on busy weekends when they opened the second window, I was the only one able to take orders there because I could do math in my head. If a meal came out to $13.56 and the customer gave me $20 I could calculate the change mentally without a register telling me how much to give back to the customer. My **work ethic** made that Burger King's numbers and drive-thru times really good. The manager treated me like I was the best thing that ever happened to him!

Some women have developed a strong **image ethic**. Their "attaboys" were *oh, you're so pretty!* or *you've got such a great little body!* They give a lot of time and attention to how they look and present themselves.

I have a beautiful friend who won Miss Virginia a couple of years ago. She is drop-dead gorgeous and she spends *a lot* of time on her image. One night, we were going out together and it literally took her two hours to get ready! I'm thinking to myself *for the love of Pete, let's go!* It would drive me crazy to spend two hours to get ready for anything! But she's in there doing her hair, her eyelashes, and the whole nine yards. I can only stand to do that a couple of times a year for special events. Here we were just going to dinner on a Friday night and she's spending hours getting ready. She spends a lot of time and energy on how good she looks and that's her image ethic.

Even for me, when I really want to look my best, there's a lot that goes into making me look good. I have to get my hair colored since I'm getting gray

165

hair now. I get my eyebrows done and I get a spray tan because I'm so, so pasty white. Without a spray tan, I look like Casper the ghost. I'm getting older now, so I need Botox for my forehead and I constantly go in for scalp treatments for the psoriasis on my scalp. These are just different things I spend a lot of time and energy on for my appearance. That's my image ethic.

When it comes to my work, nobody has to tell me to get up and go to work because I've created work habits in my life. Every Monday through Friday, even though I'm my own boss and I don't have anyone standing over my shoulder telling me what to do, I get up and go to work. If I wanted to take the entire week off I could, but I don't because my work ethic is so ingrained in who I am. My work ethic is based on the habits I've created. I get up and go to work every day, make it happen, and don't finish until it's done!

If I don't pay enough attention to my image ethic because I'm working too hard, my eating suffers. I don't take care of my image when I'm consumed with work, and I'm likely to just grab a pizza and keep it moving if my appearance is a mess.

When it comes to your **eating ethic**, overeating can create the wrong kind of momentum for the rest of your day. After you overeat, you're tired and sluggish and you can't get your work done. If you're someone who goes out and drinks every night, you're creating a habit that makes you less efficient the next day. You want to create positive **momentum habits**. These are habits that create momentum in your life. If I go to the gym first thing in the morning, that's a momentum habit because it propels me forward for the rest of the day. Exercise makes me feel better, so I'm going to be more productive. See? Momentum habits feed into the other parts of your life.

In order to create new momentum habits, you have to identify your unhealthy habits and break them. These habits begin with a trigger that kickstarts a routine and ends with a pleasure you use to satisfy your emotions.

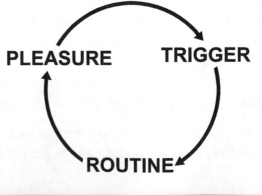

I have a trigger that activates right after lunch. If I eat too much at lunch (**trigger**), 30 minutes later my blood sugar will drop and I'll want something sweet to eat. So, I'll walk across the street to Whole Foods (**routine**) and get a piece of chocolate with almonds and eat it (**pleasure**). Now, I have this habit that every day at 2:30 I really want some chocolate.

Honestly identify the pleasure. Is it the chocolate? Is it the energy that comes from the sugar? Is it that I'm taking a break because I'm exhausted from working? Or, is it just fun? Whenever I go across the street to Whole Foods I take my friend, Heather. During that time, we get to chit-chat, talk about our day and make each other laugh. You have to identify what that pleasure is and then determine **how do I change my pleasure?**

If I'm not really hungry, then I can walk to Whole Foods and get a cup of coffee or just go to the office coffee bar and save money. If it's about spending time with my friend, I could just go along for the walk and let her buy something. I could even walk to her desk and have a cup of water or green tea. This is also a great opportunity to spend time with the Lord. Try setting an alarm for 15 minutes and see if you still want the food when that times has passed. Set the alarm a second time and see if the craving is still there.

I've told you about my routine of eating every time I walk into the house. I developed that habit when I was younger. My school served lunch so early at 11am and the meals were small. I ran around like a chicken at school and when I got home from school at 3pm I was starving and ate everything. My mom, being a healthy eater, would make gross things like turkey enchiladas with tofu for dinner. *Yuck!* Since my mom was a terrible cook, I think I felt that I needed to eat as much as I could and fill up before she got home. However, I would still eat a little something at dinner because I felt I needed to eat even though I wasn't really hungry. If she did make something that was good for dinner, I would eat all of that!

I recognized that coming home was my trigger that started the routine of snacking for the pleasure of eating. You have to realize what your trigger is and come up with a new routine. My new routine is to take a bath with Epsom salt when I first get home because that is a big pleasure for me. It lets me relax and not go crazy.

No Quitting

My mom really did a good job of instilling in me an attitude that doesn't quit. I signed up for softball when I was 12 years old because all my friends did. My first game, I hated it! I wasn't good at it and everyone else was so much better. I got hit with the ball a couple of times and I totally ran into the fence coming into home plate and got a bloody lip.

"I don't like this," I told my mom. "I quit!"

But my mom said "You are not quitting!" She never let me quit the team, and today I'm not a quitter.

If I go on a listing appointment, but don't get the property, I don't say, "That's it I'm not doing any more listings!"

It didn't work out, so what? I'm moving on to the next one.

How do you respond after one bad day of eating? Do you say, "I did terrible today and I'm just not going to do this anymore. I'm done with this. It's not working."

Suppose you have a day where you eat beyond your eating window? Fine! Get back up the next day and get right back on the plan. If you have one bad day at your job do you just quit? No! You're going to have good days and bad days but you have to keep going no matter what. The great thing is that you're not restricted on what you can eat, so you can't ever say you failed. Your only guideline is to abide by the 80/20 Rule and not overeat. Even so, if you have a day where you eat 70/30 or 50/50, pick yourself back up and start again. It's not the end of the world. You are **not** going to give up and say "this plan doesn't work for me."

I recently went out for Mexican food and they gave us chips and salsa to eat while we waited for our meals. I ate more than I should have and was feeling full by the time my meal came. I ate it anyway because that old mindset that I always have to eat what's in front of me was in my head. So, I ate too much. Do I throw away the whole plan and all of my progress over that one meal? No, I keep going!

168

Part II Conclusion

At the time that I'm writing this, it's about 11 o'clock in the morning and I haven't eaten at all since my one meal yesterday. I felt my hunger rising but I didn't want to eat just yet, so I decided to open my Bible to the book of Daniel.

> **Daniel 9:3-5 (NASB)**
> *³ So I gave my attention to the Lord God to seek Him by prayer and supplications, with fasting, sackcloth and ashes. ⁴ I prayed to the Lord my God and confessed and said, "Alas, O Lord, the great and awesome God, who keeps His covenant and loving kindness for those who love Him and keep His commandments, ⁵ we have sinned, committed iniquity, acted wickedly and rebelled, even turning aside from Your commandments and ordinances.*

The word "supplications" stood out to me in the first verse. I looked it up and learned it comes from a Latin word that means "to plead humbly." Then I started to write down the things I saw Daniel doing in this scripture and I found four:

1) He prayed
2) He fasted
3) He supplicated
4) He confessed sin

I did those four things this morning. I pleaded humbly to the Lord that He would help me through this eating challenge. In this passage, we can see what the attitude of Daniel's heart was when he fasted. He sought the Lord earnestly, and that's the attitude we should have when we fast.

169

When we deny our cravings for physical food, we're telling God, "I am craving more of you and more of Your Word. I want to read it and understand it." It's not easy. You have to really go to God and ask him to remove the blinders when you read the Word.

Pray, "God, please let me know what this means and how I can apply it to my life."

One thing people constantly ask me about The Chantel Ray Way is "What can I eat? I need an exact diet plan. I'm the type of person who needs to know exactly what to eat for breakfast, lunch, and dinner."

I see commercials for different diet plans and I think these things are a trap. Diets had me bound for many years and I finally understand how to be free. This book is designed to set you free with a totally new vision of how to eat and how food fits in your life.

This plan will work no matter what's going on in your life. People use excuses all the time to keep from getting started:

"This is a stressful time."
"My schedule is crazy."
"We're planning a vacation next week."

I don't care if it's the week before your period! This plan will work for you because you're making this decision:

I'm not going to eat because I'm tired, bored, or cranky.
I'm no longer eating for any other emotional reason.
I'm only eating when my body is physically hungry.

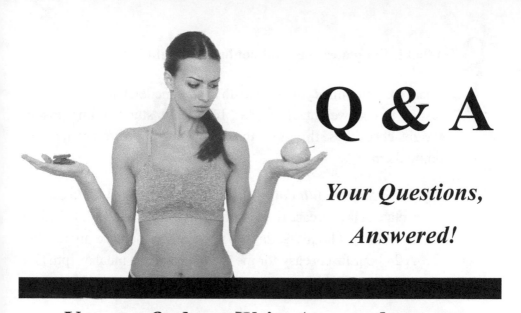

Q & A

Your Questions, Answered!

You can find my *Waist Away* podcast on iTunes and the Google Play Store. On the podcast, I answer questions from listeners about The Chantel Ray Way. I included the most commonly asked questions in the section below to help you along your journey.

Q: Do I need to always leave food on my plate? What if I'm giving myself smaller servings of food?

A: In the beginning of this journey, I think it's a good practice to leave at least one bite of food on your plate to mentally free you from bondage to food. The truth is that when you wait 20 minutes you're going to realize you're already full anyway. Practice letting go of the "clean your plate" mentality. You're learning to listen to when you're hungry and when you're full.

171

Q: What if I'm plateauing and not losing weight?

A: There are four things you need to do in conjunction with intermittent fasting to lose weight. If you feel like you're stuck and not losing weight, check these things off the list and make sure you're actually doing them.

1. *Use a Shorter Window* - One of the first things I do to escape a plateau is decrease the length of my eating window. I'll add a few more 24 hour fast days to my week to increase my results. A 24 hour fast is easy for me to do. I can eat a meal at 1pm and not eat again 1:30pm the next day; that's a 24 hour fast.

2. *Wait for Stomach Growl* - Don't lose track of getting to true hunger. Your first meal of the day should never come before your stomach growl.

3. *Eat When You're Hungry* - While you may not wait for a stomach growl to eat your second meal of the day, you should still be waiting until you're actually hungry to eat. We never eat unless we're hungry. Pay attention to your hunger scale. You should only eat your first meal at a 1 and your second meal at a 1-2.

0 - Hamster Hungry: Starving, ravenous, weak, grouchy. All you can think about is what to eat and how you can get it. You may get a headache, struggle to concentrate, or get "hangry" (hungry + angry).

1 - Stomach is Growling: Empty stomach. You can physically hear your stomach growling and feel an empty sensation. It's important that you feel both sensations because your stomach can growl for other non-hunger reasons like digestion. Be sure that it's growling because it's empty. Everything sounds good to eat at this point of hunger.

2 - Hungry: You're starting to think about food and certain things sound good to you. You're deciding what your body is craving.

3 - Not Hungry/Not Full: Neutral. You sense that there is some food in your stomach and you're at peace. Your stomach feels comfortable.

4 - Satisfied/Full: Comfortably full. You might want to eat more, but you shouldn't.

5 - Stuffed: Uncomfortably full. You're getting tired because your body is using all of its energy to digest food. You may want to take a nap or need to unbuckle your belt. You feel as if you've overeaten.

4. *No Overeating* - This is the most important factor that you have to be honest with yourself about. You can not overeat no matter what. If you're still eating too many calories you're not going to lose weight no matter how much you fast.

You should only start looking at calories after you've confirmed that you're doing those four things. Take one week to evaluate what you're eating and what amount of calories you should be consuming to lose the weight you want to lose. You might be surprised by how many calories are actually in the foods we eat. For example, there are 90 calories in just one tablespoon of peanut butter. That can add up if you're not careful.

Q: Can I be paleo as a vegetarian or vegan?

A: You can, but you're going to have very limited sources of protein. You need to eat a lot of nut butters and things like pea or hemp protein. One way to get protein is to drink smoothies.

Q: What if I'm reaching the end of my six-hour window and my stomach isn't growling? Can I eat?

A: Let's say you waited for your stomach to growl and you began your window at 12:30pm. Your window ends at 6:30pm, but maybe your stomach hasn't growled by the time your family is eating dinner at 5pm. Let's go back to that hunger scale. For the very first meal you need to be at a 1 before you start your window. At your next meal (like the 5pm family dinner), you can be a 2 and eat something really small. This way your stomach doesn't growl just after your window closes leaving you feeling tempted to eat.

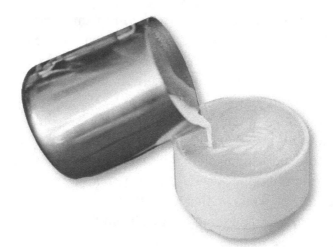

Q: What if I like to have coffee with cream in the morning?

A: If you're the kind of person who lives for their coffee with cream every morning, you're going to have to make an adjustment for a little while. It is possible to have coffee with cream and no sugar every morning and still get results. If you decide to do that, just know that you may not get results as fast as someone else. This is because you're elevating your blood sugar when you drink coffee

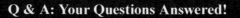

with cream. I personally recommend you don't do it. However, if that is your one hang up that's keeping you from starting this plan, then keep your coffee with cream.

Whatever you decide to do, it's best to wait and drink coffee 3-4 hours after you wake up or at least until you start getting hungry. Caffeine is an appetite suppressant, so when you drink it, it pushes you so that you can fast a little longer. On days when you're fasting but you feel like you just *have* to eat, that's when you drink the black coffee or unsweetened tea.

Q: **Once I break the seal, I get out of control. Once I have one chip, I have to have 20. Once I eat one French fry, I'm going to eat the whole thing! What if I don't know how to stop eating?**

A: The reason you're out of control is because you've deprived yourself of the foods you want and you told yourself that these are "bad foods."

Yesterday, I went to Ocean Breeze Waterpark with my family. One of them got pizza, one got a hot dog, one got french fries, and they all got ice cream. I asked my husband for one bite of his pizza and it tasted disgusting. It was like the worst thing! Then I had a french fry and I thought these are the worst fries ever! It was very easy to stop eating. The most I ate was three bites of ice cream. That goes back to the rule of decadent foods – just have a few bites.

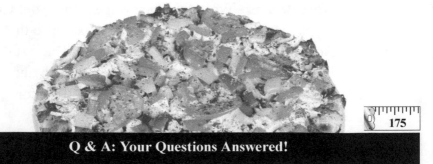

The point is this: if I didn't have that stuff I would have been sitting there thinking, *I want that pizza! I want those fries!* Instead, I had one bite of all of them and thought *eh*. I decided that the food was so disgusting that I wasn't going to eat. I wasn't starving hungry so it wasn't a problem. I've made a decision that I'm only going to fill my body with things I truly love. Why am I going to waste my calories on foods that are just *eh*.

Q: **I have low blood sugar. Can I do intermittent fasting?**

A: I have a major problem with low blood sugar. I woke up this morning not feeling well, so around 8:30 I decided to take my blood sugar. It was 63. Anything under 70 is considered low and when you're fasting your blood sugar should be between 80-100. I don't feel good when I'm in the 60-70 range. Now, I'm not a doctor and this entire book is based on my personal experiences and what works for me. This is my advice based on being a person who's had low blood sugar for a very long time. Consult your physician before doing these things.

1. *Get a monitor* - First you need to find out if you indeed have low blood sugar or if you're just constantly spiking and crashing because of a high sugar diet. Get yourself a monitor and actually test your blood sugar. If this is truly a problem for you, then you might want to eat smaller meals so that your stomach growls sooner and you can eat again.

2. *Move Around* - Typically, when you exercise your blood sugar drops but I have found in my own experience that when my blood sugar is really low and I exercise and have some caffeine it actually goes back up. Do a little research and you'll find there are other people who have a similar reaction.

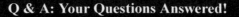

3. ***Drink unsweetened tea*** - Like I said before, I woke up this morning with my blood sugar at 63. I got up, walked around the house and drank a glass of unsweetened tea. By 11am, my blood sugar was 104 which is actually considered pre-diabetic. I went to Lucky Oyster later and had egg whites with spinach and onions as well as an egg and cheese biscuit with half of the biscuit removed. Twenty minutes after that meal, my blood sugar had only risen to 125. That's pretty good for it to only rise that much after eating a whole meal.

Unless your blood sugar is below 70, you shouldn't be eating when you're in your fasting time. Look, you're talking to the low blood sugar queen! If I can do it, so can you. You just have to check your blood sugar to see where it really is. Also, confirm you actually have a low blood sugar problem and that you aren't just addicted to sugar!

Q: **Aren't you going to eat so much more when you're in your eating window?**

A: In the beginning, I think you will. You'll have to remind yourself not to overeat. However, one of the benefits of fasting is that it gets you out of the habit of eating just because it's a certain time of day, and into the habit of eating only when you're hungry. It gets rid of the "I'm bored" snacking habit. That was a big deal for me. You have to be very careful not to eat out of boredom even if you are in your six-hour window.

Q: What should I do if I'm having really bad bouts of being "hangry?"

A: When I'm hangry (hungry and angry for those who don't know) I become a bear. One of the things that makes you hangry is your shift in ranges of blood sugar. When you're doing intermittent fasting, believe it or not, your blood sugar is more stable. I feel amazing right now - or super-duper really good as my son likes to say - so I'm going to go ahead and take my blood sugar for you guys and see what it is. I'm at 97. I feel the best when I'm fasting and my blood sugar is in the range of 90-100. It's when I'm in the 70-80 range that I'm not feeling good.

Q: What if I'm not seeing results?

A: If you're not seeing results, the first question you need to ask yourself is, "What am I drinking?" Are you drinking Diet Coke, coffee with cream, flavored water with sugar in it? These are little things that can slow your weight loss. Believe it or not, they spike your insulin and that's something you don't want to do.

Keep in mind that losing weight takes time. I didn't lose anything for the first two weeks. That's why I don't recommend weighing yourself on a scale every day. Only weigh yourself once a week and at times when you're feeling really thin. Weighing yourself every day can discourage you.

Q: Can I do this Vegan?

A: You absolutely can keep a vegan diet with this plan. You can do whatever you want as long as you're following the principles of **fasting, never overeating** and **only eating when you're hungry**. If you're trying to do 80% paleo like me, then you're going to have to eat a lot more veggies and avocados and fats.

I believe God calls different people to different things. For example, God called me to give 90% of my income and to live on 10%, but he didn't call everyone to do that. If you want to be vegan, I'm 100% on board with that. I believe the Bible is saying eat whatever you want. If you feel like God is calling you not to eat meat, who am I to say to eat meat? You have to decide what is best for you. I believe that eating meat and avoiding a whole lot of dairy and gluten is the best thing for my body.

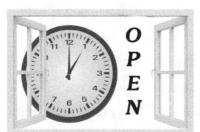
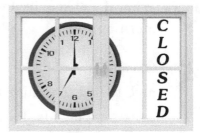

Q: How does the fasting window begin?

A: If you're having trouble figuring out the beginning of your fasting window, remember that you are free to determine when you start and stop eating. The second you start eating, you're in your **eating window** and you are considered to be in the **fed state**. Your eating window is closed the minute you stop eating and the **fasting window** begins.

I talked to a girl this weekend who told me she wakes up in the morning starving but is not a dinner person. If you're like that, you may want to do a 9am-2pm eating window. That's fine; that's your eating window. Your window is closed when you eat your very last bite.

Now, some people argue that when your fasting window begins, you're not really in a fasted state. For example, if you finished eating at 2pm, you're not immediately in a fasted state at 3pm because your body is still fueling itself off of the food you just ate. That's true, but it's not what we're talking about for the fasting window. We're dealing with the **time you're eating** vs. **the time you're fasting**. You get yourself to the fasted state by waiting until your stomach growls the next day. It's an accomplishment when your stomach growls because now you're really starting to burn fat.

Q: **What if I'm required to take food with my medication in the morning?**

A: Obviously, you'll have to break your fast in the morning, so you need to find something that will not cause your insulin to spike. Look for a high-fat food: something with cream or with a lot of butter. An egg is good as well. The yolk is very high-fat, low-carb. I would eat anything I could think of that was high-fat and low-carb, and I would eat as little of it in the morning that I could. Then I would wait for my stomach to growl before eating again. I definitely wouldn't try to have a whole meal. I wouldn't stress about it, but I would just make sure I had enough in my body so the medicine wouldn't mess up my stomach.

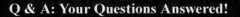

Q: What about body odor?

A: I had a friend tell me that once she started fasting she was getting more intense body odor. She said her armpits and breath smelled more. That is just a matter of your body detoxing. Use a lot of mouthwash if your breath smells bad. Carry an extra deodorant with you in your purse for your armpits. It gets better, but right now your body is trying to get used to it. It may be kind of unpleasant, but you should really look at it as something that's good. It means you're doing a good thing for your body. Also, it causes an unexpected positive side effect: more showers! If you have a problem with eating impulsively, showers and baths are really good for you. It de-stresses you. If you're having an issue with body odor, use it as an opportunity to bathe instead of eat and increase your weight loss!

Q: What if I'm not losing weight doing the eight-hour window?

A: I've found that women have a hard time losing weight if they're only doing eight hour eating windows. It's not enough fasting time and they're usually eating too much at each meal as well.

If you're working out, though, there may be another explanation. You may not be losing weight on the scale, but your body composition could be changing. Take me, for example: I am such a muscle builder. My mom used to smack me on the butt and call me the Rock of Gibraltar because I am just a solid piece of meat! There's a lot of muscle in my body. So, I have a jacket that I used to never be able to clasp both buttons, but now it fits just perfect!

I'm not seeing the results I want when I get on the scale, but these other signs let me know my body is actually changing. Ultimately, you want to change your body composition more than you want to lose weight.

Q: Are artificial sweeteners harmful?

A: Here's the bottom line: you will not get the best results if you consume artificial sweeteners. The biggest area of struggle for most people is with drinking water. I have so many friends that say they hate water. They never drink it unless it's zero-calorie flavored water. However, I believe that when you do something for a few days, you just get used to it. For example, I used to always need some sort of Splenda in my tea because I thought unsweetened tea was disgusting. Now, I can drink my tea with no sweetener at all. It's something you'll get used to.

Q: Can I have artificial sweeteners during my eating window?

A: Once you're in your eating window, you can have them as much as you want. Do I like it? No! Go back to the section on Chemical City. For me, artificial sweeteners are the Devil and I'll never eat them. I don't like the way they taste, and, if I'm going to eat something sweet, I want it to be real, live sugar. If you want to eat them, you're free to do so, but your results won't be as good.

If you'll do a web search on the effect of artificial sweeteners on blood sugar, you'll see competing results. I think it varies for every individual. Forget the studies and try it for yourself. If you're considering having artificial sweeteners in your diet, check your blood sugar before and after having them and see what happens.

Q: What do I do when I'm not getting the results I want?

A: Do more Big Power Fasts. That's my technique to step up my weight loss. I wait a little later in the day to eat, and I drink more caffeine to get me through. Sometimes I'll eat 95% paleo instead of 80/20 as well.

Q: What do I do when I go on vacation?

A: I'm going on a four-day vacation in a couple of weeks and I'm going to extend my eating windows to eight hours. If you're doing an extended vacation – like a month – I would suggest starting your window later in the day. You could do something like 1-9pm. I definitely recommend that you don't weigh yourself as soon as you get back from vacation. Like I've said before, I weigh myself when I feel skinny.

Now, if you want to continue to *lose* weight while you're on vacation and not just maintain, then stick to eating one meal a day while being lenient on the 80/20 rule. Personally, I eat less while I'm traveling because jet lag throws me off and I don't do as good a job. A note about the **enjoyment scale**: you are never going to find something at the airport that's a four. Airport food is just nasty! Even though you're on vacation, stick to 4s and 5s on the enjoyment scale. If it isn't good, just don't eat. You're going to have more fun on your vacation if you're feeling lean, so don't abandon the plan just because you're traveling. When you're on the beach in your bikini you want to feel good!

Q: Are you getting enough calories when you eat one meal a day?

A: I'm sorry, but my aunt is 89lbs and she is never worried if she's getting enough calories! You're not going to ruin your metabolism by eating one meal a day; that's a myth. You need to get this sort of thinking out of your mind. You are **not** overweight because you don't eat enough calories. Let's be real honest with ourselves. That excuse is ludicrous, and it came from the diet industry.

As always, eat when you're hungry and eat until you're satisfied on your Big Power Fast. Don't use the Big Power Fast as an excuse to get stuffed. This is very, very important.

Q: I'm not seeing my weight change on the scale. What's wrong?

A: I learned about something recently called the "whoosh effect." It explains why you don't always see a consistent change in your weight every day while you're burning fat. Because of the law of thermodynamics, burning more calories than you consume results in weight loss as your body gets the energy it needs from your fat reserves. This isn't a theory; it's actual physics. If you don't give your body food, it has to use the fat in your body. So, you may wonder why you can go a whole week and not lose weight when you know you were burning fat. That's where the "whoosh effect" comes in. It has to do with water retention. The idea is that your fat cells become filled with water as you're burning fat. Because of this, the scale doesn't change even though you did in fact burn fat. However, once your body finally drops that water (maybe 1-2 weeks later or more depending on the person) you lose a bunch of weight at once. That's called the "whoosh effect[5]" It's like the sound of your pounds being flushed down the toilet. Get it? It's not that you actually lost that many pounds overnight. It's that your weight loss finally "caught up" with your fat loss.

[5] Muir, Chris, "How Whooshes Impact Your Weight Loss"
http://leanmuscleproject.com/how-whooshes-impact-your-weight-loss/
Shellabarger, Brian. "The 'Whoosh' Effect" http://100down.org/the-whoosh-effect/
"Of Whooshes and Squishy Fat" http://www.bodyrecomposition.com/fat-loss/of-whooshes-and-squishy-fat.html/

Q & A: Your Questions Answered!

I lost no weight at all during my first two weeks of doing this plan. My third week I lost six pounds and my fourth week I lost four. **WHOOSH!** I lost all this weight! That's why I don't like getting on the scale every day. You're getting yourself worked up for no reason. Here's what I suggest as a better way to measure your weight loss: get a pair of pants that you don't ever wash or dry and try them on regularly to see how you're progressing. I even prefer this method to measuring your inches with measuring tape. When you use measuring tape, you have to be sure to measure the same exact spot and pull the tape just right every time or your reading won't be accurate.

Q: I'm doing intermittent fasting and now I don't feel good?

A: Don't make the mistake of overdosing on the wrong foods just because you're allowed to eat whatever you want now. I've seen a lot of people who were eating really clean but then went the complete opposite direction when they started intermittent fasting. Your body isn't going to feel well if you do that. This is why I focus on eating clean foods even if they're not "healthy." I know I have a high fat diet. I don't worry about fat. I eat nuts that are high in fat, steak with butter and all that stuff because the more fat I eat the better I feel. It's chemicals that I stay away from because I like to feel my best.

Q: How do I know if I'm getting enough nutrients in my body?

A: I take a lot of vitamins because I feel like the food we eat doesn't have as much as I need. Visit chantelrayway.com/vitamins.

Q: What are your thoughts on having a cheat meal?

A: I don't call it a cheat meal because I eat what I want every day. On days that I'm not feeling great, I fill my body with super healthy foods to get my energy up.

Right now, I'm craving Baker's Crust's Gotta Have It burger. Since I want to keep it clean today, I'm going to take away the bun and wrap it in lettuce. When I need a lot of energy, I don't eat as many carbs. I'll eat red meat because my iron levels are lower than the average Joe. So, I'm going to have this burger wrapped in lettuce with some fries for potassium, and that will be my one meal for the day.

Q: What are your thoughts on alcohol and wine?

A: I went to a pool party last night and someone asked me if I wanted champagne. I told her no because I don't like to drink my calories. I have a ton of friends that do intermittent fasting and they really like to drink. I believe the Bible says that Jesus drank wine, and I believe drinking is fine as long as you don't get drunk. There are also health benefits to drinking red wine. I'm a proponent of drinking wine if the Holy Spirit leads you to. I'm just not a drinker. I probably drink two times a year and I don't love it. I actually have this mental block to drinking because of all my years of dieting. It's this thought that if I don't drink my calories, I can have more to eat. I have plenty of friends that are very skinny and would much rather drink their calories than eat them. The main thing is that, if you're drinking, you're doing it during your eating window.

Q: **But doesn't alcohol make you gain weight?**

A: I have this group called the Thursday Funday group. A lot of them are not Christians, but I absolutely adore them. I look at how much they eat and drink and they definitely increase their calories with alcohol. However, they are still as thin as they can be. Keep in mind most of those girls only eat one meal a day and maybe a snack. Most of them don't start eating before two or three in the afternoon, and they stay in that six or eight-hour window. Keep looking at the line between eating and overeating. If you are eating and drinking in your window, the alcohol should be fine.

Q: **What are the benefits of red wine?**

A: There are all kinds of studies explaining why you should drink red wine. They say it regulates your blood sugar. I don't really know because I don't drink it, but if Jesus drank it I'm not going to look at you negatively for doing it. If you want to be literal I suppose you could say you drink it to be more like Him. HAHA!

Q: **How strict do I have to be on the 80/20?**

A: The 80/20 is important. It's 100% clean eating that I don't recommend. Yesterday, I had nothing but grilled veggies, grilled shrimp, and salad. However, I ate a large volume of food and I ate so clean because I was surrounded by people who were eating that way too. I really wanted a potato and pasta and I should have gotten that. I could have done that and only eaten a few bites. Instead, I tried to do 100% clean and ended up feeling deprived. So, when I got home I went a half hour over my eating window and ate a bite

187

of pudding and ten mini peanut butter Ritz crackers. That was a mini-binge for me. When I try to be perfect with my eating, I get in a bad place and lose control a little bit. When I eat what I want in the 80/20 system, it doesn't affect my body negatively. You want to make clean choices, but you don't want to overdo it. Not overeating is the #1 thing.

Q: What's the ideal number of times to poop?

A: Most of the people I talk to feel their best when they have 2-3 bowel movements a day. At that number, you're cleaning out your gut and getting rid of toxins in your body. Keep in mind that if you're eating only one meal a day then you're probably going to be running to the bathroom less.

I've done a lot of study on gut health and I think it's one of the most important things for you to work on. Your bowel movements are influenced by what time you're eating and by something called the **gut microbiome**. The healthier your microbiome, the better your digestive system will work. What tears up your microbiome is eating too much processed food. When your gut is out of balance you have inflammation, excess fat, and insulin resistance. If you find yourself feeling constipated a lot, you can take probiotics to clean out your gut. I take between 100-180 million probiotics every day but it can be very expensive.

Candida – or yeast infection – can give you chronic fatigue, digestive problems, bloating and more. While cutting down on sugar in your diet can help stop the overgrowth, candida actually makes you crave sugar more! Avoid these kinds of conditions and stick to your 80/20.

I've seen some people say they have runny stool or constipation from intermittent fasting. If you have problems with constipation, magnesium can be good for you. You can take it in powder or oil form. You also need to look at how much fiber you have in your diet. I don't think the American diet includes very much fiber, so I take a fiber supplement every day.

Q: Should I be eating low-carb?

A: I try not to focus on eating a low-carb diet. Even if you cut down your carbohydrate intake, you could still easily eat 3,000-4,000 calories in a day. I've seen people actually gain weight on a low-carb diet because the foods they were eating were high in fat. My answer to how to eat is always this: eat in your window and never overeat. You shouldn't be counting calories and you shouldn't be counting carbs. Eat high-quality, real foods, eat only when you're hungry, and stop eating when you're full.

Q: How do I decide the length of my eating window each day?

A: It depends on your schedule and what you have going on. For example, I have company at my house today, so I sat down with them when they were eating breakfast but I didn't eat with them. I'd rather skip breakfast because that's easier for me than lunch and dinner. Since I still need to maintain my six-hour window, I'm going to eat from 1-7pm so I can have that meal time with my visitors. Although it's better to use the same timeframe for your eating window every day, you can make adjustments on the fly depending on your schedule and how you feel.

Q: When does my window begin? Do I track my eating or do I track my fasting?

A: In this book, we track our eating with eating windows. Alternatively, you can choose to track the number of hours you fast instead of with a fasting window. Your eating window begins as soon as you consume your first calorie for the day, and it ends when you consume your last calorie. A fasting window begins after your last calorie of the day and ends when you consume your first calorie. For advice on tracking, visit chantelrayway.com/tracking.

Q: What if I want to have a beer while watching football on a Sunday night but I finished eating earlier at 7pm?

A: When that last drop of beer is consumed, that's when you've begun fasting. You have to count that beer. If you are consuming drink or food, then you are still in your eating window, no exceptions.

Q: How do I decide the length of my eating window each day?

A: We have a calendar (see Principle 3) to get you started, but ultimately this is individualized in the long-term. Men seem to do better with 14 or 16 hour fasts (10 or 8 hour eating windows) and women do better with 20 or 18 hour fasts (4 or 6 hour eating windows). Personally, I like to do 4 hour eating windows two or three times a week.

Q: How obsessive should I be on the eating window? If I started my window at 12:06pm, do I have to close it at exactly 6:06pm?

A: Don't get obsessive! You don't have to pinpoint it to the exact minute. What you want is a consistent window to help you develop a routine, but this should never be stressful. Intermittent fasting is a tool that takes the stress out of your eating. If you start getting obsessive, then you're on the wrong track.

Q: If my eating window just opened, but I'm not truly hungry should I eat anyway?

A: No. If you're trying to lose weight, you definitely don't need to be forcing yourself to eat. Remember, we eat when we're truly hungry.

Q: I've read before that you should eat before you get hungry to avoid binging. Is that true?

A: If your car doesn't need gas, you don't put gas in it. If your bill isn't due, you don't pay money on it. I believe the same principle should apply to our bodies. I get the idea of trying to avoid binging, and, honestly, the first couple of weeks of intermittent fasting you'll probably overeat some. However, you will adjust.

Q: What are some tips to not overeat on your first meal of the day? Sometimes my work schedule is so busy that I can't take a break to eat. When I do finally begin my eating window, I'm starving.

A: Stay away from simple carbs and sugars on your first meal. Keep your digestion in mind and eat slowly. You're going to be full 20 minutes before you realize it, so don't rush through your meal just because you're hungry. Another great tip is to drink a glass of water an hour before you eat. This will take the edge off of the hunger so you can sit down and enjoy your meal without overeating. In fact, whenever you're feeling overwhelmed by hunger throughout the day, try drinking water. If it's been 45 minutes since your last drink, you could actually be dehydrated. Don't drink a ton of water while you're eating, though. You might dilute your stomach acids and hinder digestion.

Q: I'm so tired after eating my first meal of the day. Why am I so exhausted from fasting?

A: Are you eating too much? What are you eating? It's more likely that what you're eating is the source of the problem rather than the fasting. If you're eating whole, clean foods I have a hard time believing you're constantly tired.

Q: I don't have enough energy to workout in my fasted state.

A: There are a lot of possibilities. Are you getting enough of all of your proteins, carbs, and fats? Are you getting enough sleep? Maybe switch your workout time to be closer to your eating window so you can eat right after. Or, eat right before. I personally like to work out fasted, but everyone is different.

Q: Are you allowed to lift heavy weights while fasting?

A: I lift heavy weights every single morning in a fasted state. I've lifted heavier weights fasted than men in my gym! My trainer, Chris Sykes, tells me he does all of the same workouts he did before he started intermittent fasting and he hasn't lost any steam.

Q: Can you still build muscle with intermittent fasting?

A: Yes. Nothing changes. If you need to get in a certain number of macros every day, you can still do that just in an eating window. You don't have to choose between the two. A lot of people who want to build muscle hear that you need to eat no more than 30 minutes after your workout to get the benefits from your food. While it's true that your cells can take in more of what you eat within 30 minutes of your workout, that's not the only time. You can eat 20-30 hours after and still get the benefits from your food.

193

Q: How do I decide on the length of my eating window? Should I be eating whole meals or half meals?

A: You have to figure out what works for you because everyone is different and our windows won't all be the same. There are some people who only eat one meal a day (also called OMAD). Some people eat in a five-hour window and have one snack and one meal a little while later. If you're someone who's going to do OMAD, just be sure you're not binging. You may need to spend time practicing it until you regulate.

Personally, I couldn't lose weight in an eight-hour window. I don't believe many women can unless you're eating really clean, really small portions. When I'm trying to maintain my weight I do a six-hour window with one medium sized meal around 12pm, and something small around 5:30pm. That works really well for me. When my goal is to lose weight, I try to stick to that one meal a day. It's usually in a four-hour window where I'm eating a nice meal that gets me to a four on the hunger scale, and then I may have another small snack. You'll need to tinker with your window to find out what works for you. If your goal is weight loss, you may need to tighten your window and the amount of food you eat. If you're maintaining, you have more flexibility. Some people want a rigid plan with someone telling them exactly what to do, but with the Chantel Ray Way, you have to modify everything to fit you.

Something you want to pay attention to is your satiety signals. It's a signal your nervous system gets that gives you that sense of fullness. Now that I'm doing intermittent fasting, my **satiety signals** are so good. Yesterday, I went to lunch and I tried a lot of different foods; I had a little bit of this and a little bit of that, and, when I was done, I was 100% satisfied with no desire to eat anything else for the rest of the day.

Q: I want to try intermittent fasting, but I have low blood sugar. Can I go that long without eating?

A: The crazy thing is intermittent fasting will actually help regulate your blood sugar. If you hang in there, you'll notice it gets better. If you begin Intermittent Fasting while having blood sugar issues, you'll need to do a good job of gradually weaning yourself off of a long eating window. You may have to start with a 12 hour eating window, then step it down to 11, then 10, and so on. I had low blood sugar as well, so I absolutely understand what it's like. Intermittent fasting's effect on blood sugar is really fascinating.

Q: How do you know when your body starts using fat storage for fuel?

A: You'll never really know the exact moment your body is attacking your fat, but I like to use my stomach growl as a general gauge. That's why I like to wait a couple of hours after I hear my stomach growl to eat. I feel like it's when my stomach starts growling that my body is out of food and starts using my fat for fuel. There's a chance that it's all just mental, but I love that feeling of my body eating away at my fat; I like to prolong that for as long as I can.

Q: Why not do a calorie restricted diet?

A: Trying to manage the total number of calories you need to eat for weight loss is too restrictive. We want to stop counting calories, stop focusing on food, and do away with the restrictions. Instead of listening to a program, we're listening to our bodies. God wired our bodies to tell us exactly what we need. We should be able to eat what our bodies crave in the amount that it needs and be satisfied. We are never going to tell you that you have to eat this or that. What's optimal, though, is the 80/20 rule.

195

Q: What should I do when I go out and everyone else is eating except me?

A: I went to dinner with friends just the other night. I had already eaten a big lunch and I wasn't hungry, so I didn't eat or drink any calories. Guess what happened? I had a fantastic time! Eating and drinking is not the only point of hanging out with friends! I had fun just sipping on water and club soda. I was able to talk more and have deeper conversations with my friends. All it takes is a mental adjustment. You can even have fun with it! When the waitress asked me what I wanted I responded, "Oh, I'm not eating. I've got to keep this skinny body of mine." That got a laugh out of everybody!

If you have real friends, they won't pressure you non-stop to eat. If someone is trying to push you to eat, just say something like, "I appreciate it, but I didn't come here to eat. I came to enjoy my time with you." Let your friends know that their understanding will help you achieve your goals the same way you help them achieve theirs.

Q: I've already lost 10 pounds! Now that I've reached my goal, should I continue intermittent fasting or stop?

A: Continue! Do it to maintain and do it because intermittent fasting has so many benefits beyond weight loss. It's a positive lifestyle change, and, personally, I can't imagine going back. There are plenty of stories of the hormonal and brain benefits of intermittent fasting people have experienced. Read Principle 3 for more on the benefits of intermittent fasting.

Q: Is intermittent fasting good for thyroid issues?

A: Always check with your doctor before you start a new diet plan. My personal experience has been stellar! I was taking 115mg of Synthroid when I started this journey because my thyroid wasn't functioning well at all. Now, I've weaned myself off of it completely.

One note about my thyroid improvement is that I also eat paleo for the 80% of my 80/20. I believe that this combination with intermittent fasting has had a huge impact on my thyroid improvement.

Now, this isn't about the thyroid, but my trainer, Chris, suffered from ankle pain for a long time from a surgery for a previous injury. He used to have pain five days out of the week, but now he's pain-free. He doesn't even need a leg brace when he plays sports anymore.

**For more information on thyroid health,
go to: www.ChantelRayWay.com/thyroid**

Q: **I'm really confused. All of my trainers have always told me that eating 5-6 small meals a day will keep my metabolism elevated. Is intermittent fasting bad for my metabolism?**

A: That claim about eating 5-6 meals a day is a myth. Your metabolic rate is not based on how many meals you eat. It's based on what type of foods you eat, your digestive health, how much you exercise, and what body type you have. For example, if I eat 6 meals of pancakes and fast food burgers, I'm not going to have a six pack. Intermittent fasting is not bad for your metabolism. Intermittent fasting has gotten me results while eating 5-6 meals a day in the past hasn't.

Q: I can only train in the morning before work. Should I eat after? How do I handle this?

A: Ideally, you want to take in protein and carbs after your workout. Post-workout, your cells are open and more of the good stuff can get in. However, not eating immediately after your workout isn't a death sentence to results. I work out in the morning and don't eat until 1 or 2pm. My trainer, Chris, usually doesn't eat until six hours after his workout. However, if you find yourself dragging during the day, then maybe that isn't for you; move your eating window to accommodate your body.

Q: Should I shift the time of day I have my eating window so my body doesn't get used to it?

A: Having your eating window at the same time every day won't really affect your metabolism. The length of the window has a greater effect. You can mix up the length of your eating windows each week to keep your metabolism from getting used to a pattern. For example, one week you might alternate each day between six and eight-hour eating windows. The next week you might throw in three Big Power Fasts. Your body does adapt to changes quickly, so mixing up the length of your eating windows is a good idea

Q: Is intermittent fasting bad for my blood sugar?

A: If you've read this far, then you already know that answer to that! One of the biggest benefits of intermittent fasting is the positive effects it has on blood sugar. Keeping insulin from being introduced to your system for 18-24 hours helps you burn fat and keep your weight down. Always check with your doctor before you start a new diet, but I've learned that much of the time people don't experience low blood sugar as often as they think. Sometimes people are just fatigued and it's because of something other than low blood sugar. My blood sugar is more stable now than it was when I was eating foods with a low glycemic index.

Q: I love having wine at 8 or 9pm after putting the kids to bed. How can I still have my wine at night?

A: Time your eating window so that it closes after your drink. If it's a six-hour window day, maybe eat from 3:30-9:30pm. If you need to have an eight-hour window to be able to have your wine, you can do that. Just remember that for women, an eight-hour window is not very effective for losing weight unless you're eating very clean, very small portions for every meal.

Q: Is intermittent fasting safe for women?

A: Well, I am a woman so...yes! Women respond to fasting differently than men because we have different hormones. For example, when I first started fasting, my menstrual cycle was 20 days late. I've read reports of this kind of thing happening for the first couple of months of fasting, but usually it returns to normal. Fasting is perfectly safe for women barring any specific medical issues you discuss with your doctor.

Q: I'm a Type 2 diabetic, and I have been off of medication and on a LCHF (low carb high fat) diet for eight months. When I try fasting for multiple days, my blood sugar drops to the low 60s. I've been taught this range is too low and it means I need to have food. Is this drop a normal short-term effect?

A: Your blood sugar will be lower while fasting, but it shouldn't be low to the point of affecting you negatively. I think maybe the combination of fasting and the LCHF might be too much. You could try cycling in higher carb days, but that's a guess without seeing the foods you're eating. Again, always check with your doctor if your blood sugar is running too low.

Q: I am brand new to intermittent fasting and I miss my wine. Is it okay to drink in my eating window?

A: You can definitely drink wine in your eating window! Just be careful to notice the sugar content in what you're drinking. There's a lot more sugar in wine than most people realize. There are also 70-80 additives in wine that you wouldn't know about without reading the contents. Find natural wines that are low in sugar. After you drink, watch your eating activity because you can start getting cravings that have nothing to do with true hunger. You don't want your eating to take a nosedive after you drink!

Q: Can I break my fast with alcohol?

A: You should break your fast with some sort of protein. Alcohol on an empty stomach isn't a great idea. Alcohol, like other high sugar drinks, can spike your insulin very harshly if you drink it at the start of your window.

Q: Can I eat a ketogenic diet with intermittent fasting and still drink alcohol?

A: The ketogenic diet is a very low-carb, high-fat diet. It's designed to keep you burning fat for energy instead of glucose. Like I've said before, alcohol has a lot of sugar. Consider losing the mixers to cut out some of those carbs. Most pure spirits are low carb; the mixers are what rack up the calories.

Q: Does drinking alcohol completely halt my fat burning?

A: No. Like anything else you eat, it's all about the nutritional value of what you're drinking. Beyond that, there's nothing inherent in alcohol that makes it more restrictive to fat burning than any other food with the same nutritional content. My thin friends use sugar-free mixers with vodka and tequila and love to drink all the time. It hasn't affected their ability to burn fat or maintain their weight.

Q: Is there a certain caloric intake I should have with intermittent fasting? Is there such a thing as too few calories? Some days I'm just ravenous!

A: How many calories you consume depends on your goals. If you're trying to lose weight and you haven't been getting strong results, then you might need to decrease your calorie intake. Of course, if you want to gain weight then you're going to need more. There is such a thing as too few calories. You can't go three weeks eating only 500 calories a day. My desire is that you learn to listen to your body. If you're a person who exercises, some days you're going to work out harder and your body is going to be hungrier. Listen to your body and eat. Eating is not a bad thing. Overeating is.

Q: I'm really concerned about doing intermittent fasting because I have low blood sugar. I'm afraid I'll pass out.

A: First, you need to determine if you actually have low blood sugar. If it's just a fatigued feeling and not a doctor's diagnosis, it's probably what you're eating that makes you feel lethargic. If you eat a huge, carb-heavy lunch, it'll raise your blood sugar so high that when it comes back down, you "crash." Adjusting how you eat is important. More protein and less carbs is how I like to eat with intermittent fasting. Also, getting fiber into your meals will help your digestion so your body isn't working overtime and making you tired while it's digesting food.

Q: **I always heard about calories in vs calories out. If I'm watching my calories, does it matter what I eat? Is there a difference between eating 1800 calories throughout the day versus eating 1800 calories in a 6-8 hour window?**

A: I believe you would be leaner in the window because of the insulin response in your body. If you're eating all day, you're filling up your glycogen cells, and, at the end of the day, they're being stored as fat. When you eat in a window, however, your insulin is turned off for the rest of the day and you burn the glycogen and get to fat burning mode faster.

Q: **Does this diet include a vegan option? If it doesn't, I'm not trying it. If it's not vegan, it can't be healthy!**

A: As long as you're following these other rules, you can be vegan if you want to be. This isn't a diet per se, so you can eat whatever you normally eat and that includes vegan. Genesis 9 makes it clear you can eat meat, but if you feel you need to eat vegan, then that is perfectly fine. The Bible tells us to be tolerant toward each other in what we eat (Romans 14:5).

Q: I've been told I have to eat carbs before working out. So, is it safe to exercise during my fasting window?

A: Your body stores a lot of glucose and carbs. If you had carbs the night before working out, then you could still have enough to get you through your workout the next morning. Personally, I'm always in a fasted state when I exercise and I'm always fine. When you're in a fasted state your endurance and stamina can actually increase. My trainer, Chris, believed the same myth about having to eat before exercising and was surprised to discover that once he started intermittent fasting he actually had more focus and stamina.

Q: I typically eat a high protein meal after my morning workout, but I want to start my eating window later in the day. Should I start skipping my post-workout meal?

A: I haven't eaten anything post-workout since I started doing intermittent fasting. When you're intermittent fasting, your workouts are going to primarily be fueled by fat and that's a good thing. It's true that, post-workout, your cells are more open to absorbing protein, but that window of time can be as long as 36 hours. You don't have to eat immediately after your workout to take advantage of that benefit.

Q: What is the longest amount of time that it's safe to fast? I'm going on vacation in less than a month and I want to speed up my weight loss.

A: 24-36 hour fasts are ideal. Anything longer than 48 hours is something your body might not be prepared for. However, it sounds like you're trying to rush for a short term goal. Don't overdo it! A couple of 24 hour fasts a week are a good way to kick up your weight loss.

Q: I'm pregnant and already freaking out about my post-baby body. Is it safe for me to start intermittent fasting while pregnant?

A: This is something you'll want to talk about with your doctor. I would've been fine fasting during my pregnancy because I would have still made sure to get in all of my nutrients. Remember that intermittent fasting isn't about restricting what you eat, but about changing the timing of when you eat. Still, fasting does affect your hormones and you want to be sure you don't do anything to affect the baby negatively, so talk to your doctor.

Q: I always wake up starving in the morning. Could I eat dinner and breakfast, but just skip lunch?

A: Unless you're someone who works a night shift, this would be hard to do. You wouldn't be able to ever have a long enough fasting window to maximize the benefits. If you're waking up starving, maybe adjust your window so that you're eating closer to your bedtime. Try drinking coffee and plenty of water to help suppress your appetite.

Q: Can I drink my coffee with MCT or coconut oil or does that break my fast?

A: I'm a big fan of both oils. My blood sugar goes down when I drink them. Now, these oils have calories and I would prefer you fast without consuming any calories. However, if this is the only way you can get through your fast, then this is the second best way. It wouldn't sabotage the entire fast. Ingesting pure fat or oil doesn't spike your insulin and MCT oil requires little digestion. If you're going to eat something, this is the best option.

Q: Can I eat some low-carb foods during my fasting window to take the edge off? They're healthy right?

A: The nutritional content of the food doesn't matter. If you're taking in calories, you're breaking the fast. If you're new to this and struggling, maybe you're fasting too long. Back it down if you have to and work your way up.

Q: How much water do you recommend I drink during my fast?

A: If you're thirsty then drink. If you're not, then you don't need to be guzzling water. You can dilute the stomach acids needed to digest food when you drink too much water. Drink just as much as you need and no more.

Q: My breath smells really bad when I fast. Is this normal?

A: It could be related to the fasting. Fasting encourages detoxification in your gut and that can have smelly effects on your breath. If you're eating a lot of protein in your diet, your body could be going into ketosis and that can cause bad breath. Try taking peppermint oil to fix the smell.

Q: Should I stop fasting if I feel shaky?

A: Check your blood sugar if you're physically shaking. It could be different things but that's a good place to start.

Q: I heard I should break my fast with protein but I recently learned meat spikes your insulin. What's the deal?

A: I was surprised to discover this, but, yes, meat can spike your insulin.

Q: I learned about the food pyramid when I was young. Are those principles still true?

A: NO! We now know that the food pyramid is not based on nutritional value. When you're eating, you need to decide what's good and what works for you. They used to say we should drink 3 cups of milk a day decades ago, but now we know that's not the best for you.

Q: I think I'm ready to try out my first 4 hour eating window. Should I eat breakfast, lunch, or dinner?

A: That's a matter of personal preference. Don't try to force yourself to eat at a certain time of day you're not comfortable with. Fasting for 20 hours is challenging enough on its own.

Q: I've been hearing a lot about the importance of gut health.

A: The process of digesting food is what they're talking about. The gut microbiome has a lot to do with how you feel. When your gut health is off, you're not digesting your food and nutrients correctly. You can have what are basically pounds of feces sitting in the lower part of your stomach. If you struggle with digesting food well, you can take digestive enzymes.

Scripture References

Proverbs 23:2 (NIV) — *and put a knife to your throat if you are given to gluttony.*

Ezekiel 16:49 (NLT) — *Sodom's sins were pride, gluttony, and laziness, while the poor and needy suffered outside her door.*

Proverbs 23:20-21 (NASB) — *Do not be with heavy drinkers of wine, Or with gluttonous eaters of meat; For the heavy drinker and the glutton will come to poverty, And drowsiness will clothe one with rags.*

Deuteronomy 21:18-21 (NASB) — *"If any man has a stubborn and rebellious son who will not obey his father or his mother, and when they chastise him, he will not even listen to them, then his father and mother shall seize him, and bring him out to the elders of his city at the gateway of his hometown. They shall say to the elders of his city, 'This son of ours is stubborn and rebellious, he will not obey us, he is a glutton and a drunkard.' Then all the men of his city shall stone him to death; so you shall remove the evil from your midst, and all Israel will hear of it and fear.*

Acts 26:18 (NASB) — *to open their eyes so that they may turn from darkness to light and from the dominion of Satan to God, that they may receive forgiveness of sins and an inheritance among those who have been sanctified by faith in Me.*

Psalm 63:5 (NLT)

⁵ You satisfy me more than the richest feast. I will praise you with songs of joy.

Ephesians 6:12 (NIV)

For our struggle is not against flesh and blood, but against the rulers, against the authorities, against the powers of this dark world and against the spiritual forces of evil in the heavenly realms.

Matthew 6:16-18 (NIV)

"When you fast, do not look somber as the hypocrites do, for they disfigure their faces to show others they are fasting. Truly I tell you, they have received their reward in full. But when you fast, put oil on your head and wash your face, so that it will not be obvious to others that you are fasting, but only to your Father, who is unseen; and your Father, who sees what is done in secret, will reward you.

Colossians 3:16a (NLT)

¹⁶ Let the message about Christ, in all its richness, fill your lives....

Matthew 4:1-2 (NIV)

4 Then Jesus was led by the Spirit into the wilderness to be tempted by the devil. ² After fasting forty days and forty nights, he was hungry.

Acts 14:23 (NIV)

²³ Paul and Barnabas appointed elders for them in each church and, with prayer and fasting, committed them to the Lord, in whom they had put their trust.

Nehemiah 1:3-4 (NIV)   *³ They said to me, "Those who survived the exile and are back in the province are in great trouble and disgrace. The wall of Jerusalem is broken down, and its gates have been burned with fire."*

⁴ When I heard these things, I sat down and wept. For some days I mourned and fasted and prayed before the God of heaven.

Ezra 8:21, 23 (NIV)   *²¹ There, by the Ahava Canal, I proclaimed a fast, so that we might humble ourselves before our God and ask him for a safe journey for us and our children, with all our possessions. ²³ So we fasted and petitioned our God about this, and he answered our prayer.*

Jonah 3:4-5,10 (NIV)   *¹ Jonah began by going a day's journey into the city, proclaiming, "Forty more days and Nineveh will be overthrown."*

⁵ The Ninevites believed God. A fast was proclaimed, and all of them, from the greatest to the least, put on sackcloth.

¹⁰ When God saw what they did and how they turned from their evil ways, he relented and did not bring on them the destruction he had threatened.

Luke 2:37 (NIV)   *³⁷ and then was a widow until she was eighty-four. She never left the temple but worshiped night and day, fasting and praying.*

Judges 20:26-30,35 (NIV)

²⁶ Then all the Israelites, the whole army, went up to Bethel, and there they sat weeping before the LORD. They fasted that day until evening and presented burnt offerings and fellowship offerings to the LORD. ²⁷ And the Israelites inquired of the LORD. (In those days the ark of the covenant of God was there, ²⁸ with Phinehas son of Eleazar, the son of Aaron, ministering before it.) They asked, "Shall we go up again to fight against the Benjamites, our fellow Israelites, or not?"

The LORD responded, "Go, for tomorrow I will give them into your hands."

²⁹ Then Israel set an ambush around Gibeah. ³⁰They went up against the Benjamites on the third day and took up positions against Gibeah as they had done before.

³⁵ The LORD defeated Benjamin before Israel, and on that day the Israelites struck down 25,100 Benjamites, all armed with swords.

Isaiah 58:4 (NIV)

⁴ Your fasting ends in quarreling and strife, and in striking each other with wicked fists.
You cannot fast as you do today and expect your voice to be heard on high.

Isaiah 58:5a (NIV)

⁵ Is this the kind of fast I have chosen only a day for people to humble themselves?

2 Corinthians 12:8-9a (NIV)

8 Three times I pleaded with the Lord to take it away from me. 9 But he said to me, "My grace is sufficient for you, for my power is made perfect in weakness."

3 John 2 (NIV)

2 Dear friend, I pray that you may enjoy good health and that all may go well with you, even as your soul is getting along well.

Exodus 15:26 (NIV)

26 He said, "If you listen carefully to the Lord your God and do what is right in his eyes, if you pay attention to his commands and keep all his decrees, I will not bring on you any of the diseases I brought on the Egyptians, for I am the Lord, who heals you."

1 Samuel 1:19-20 (NIV)

19 Early the next morning they arose and worshiped before the Lord and then went back to their home at Ramah. Elkanah made love to his wife Hannah, and the Lord remembered her. 20 So in the course of time Hannah became pregnant and gave birth to a son. She named him Samuel, saying, "Because I asked the Lord for him."

Galatians 5:17 (NIV)

17 For the flesh desires what is contrary to the Spirit, and the Spirit what is contrary to the flesh. They are in conflict with each other, so that you are not to do whatever you want.

Matthew 6:17-18 (NIV)

17 But when you fast, put oil on your head and wash your face, 18 so that it will not be obvious to others that you are fasting, but only to your Father, who is unseen; and your Father, who sees what is done in secret, will reward you.

Matthew 9:15 (NIV)	*15 Jesus answered, "How can the guests of the bridegroom mourn while he is with them? The time will come when the bridegroom will be taken from them; then they will fast.*
Proverbs 25:16 (NIV)	*16 If you find honey, eat just enough— too much of it, and you will vomit.*
Proverbs 23:21 (MSG)	*Drunks and gluttons will end up on skid row, in a stupor and dressed in rags.*
Proverbs 25:27 (NLT)	*27 It's not good to eat too much honey, and it's not good to seek honors for yourself.*
Exodus 34:14 (NLT)	*You must worship no other gods, for the Lord, whose very name is Jealous, is a God who is jealous about his relationship with you.*
Exodus 20:1-6 (MSG)	*God spoke all these words:* *I am God, your God, who brought you out of the land of Egypt, out of a life of slavery.* *No other gods, only me.* *No carved gods of any size, shape, or form of anything whatever, whether of things that fly or walk or swim. Don't bow down to them and don't serve them because I am God, your God...*
Exodus 32:2-4 (MSG)	*So Aaron told them, "Take off the gold rings from the ears of your wives and sons and daughters and bring them to me." They all did it; they removed the gold rings from their ears and brought them to Aaron. He took the gold from their hands and cast it in the form of a calf, shaping it with an engraving tool.*

*The people responded with enthusiasm: "These
are your gods, O Israel, who brought you up from
Egypt!"*

Isaiah 44:9 (NLT)

*⁹ How foolish are those who manufacture idols.
These prized objects are really worthless.
The people who worship idols don't know this, so
they are all put to shame.*

**1 Corinthians 3:16
(NIV)**

*¹⁶ Don't you know that you yourselves are God's
temple and that God's Spirit dwells in your midst?*

Hebrews 12:2 (NIV)

*fixing our eyes on Jesus, the pioneer and perfecter
of faith. For the joy set before him he endured the
cross, scorning its shame, and sat down at the right
hand of the throne of God.*

Romans 12:1 (NIV)

*Therefore, I urge you, brothers and sisters, in view
of God's mercy, to offer your bodies as a living
sacrifice, holy and pleasing to God—this is your
true and proper worship.*

Psalm 16:11 (NIV)

*You make known to me the path of life; you will
fill me with joy in your presence, with eternal
pleasures at your right hand.*

**1 Corinthians 10:31
(NIV)**

*³¹ So whether you eat or drink or whatever you
do, do it all for the glory of God.*

**Colossians 2:20-23
(NIV)**

*²⁰ Since you died with Christ to the elemental
spiritual forces of this world, why, as though you
still belonged to the world, do you submit to its
rules: ²¹ "Do not handle! Do not taste! Do not*

touch!"? 22 These rules, which have to do with things that are all destined to perish with use, are based on merely human commands and teachings. 23 Such regulations indeed have an appearance of wisdom, with their self-imposed worship, their false humility and their harsh treatment of the body, but they lack any value in restraining sensual indulgence.

Acts 3:1 (NIV)

19 Repent, then, and turn to God, so that your sins may be wiped out, that times of refreshing may come from the Lord,

Hebrews 3:7-11 (MSG)

Today, please listen; don't turn a deaf ear as in "the bitter uprising," that time of wilderness testing! Even though they watched me at work for forty years, your ancestors refused to let me do it my way; over and over they tried my patience. And I was provoked, oh, so provoked! I said, "They'll never keep their minds on God; they refuse to walk down my road." Exasperated, I vowed, "They'll never get where they're going, never be able to sit down and rest."

Ecclesiastes 6:7 (NIV)

7 Everyone's toil is for their mouth, yet their appetite is never satisfied.

Joel 2:26 (NIV)

26 You will have plenty to eat, until you are full, and you will praise the name of the Lord your God, who has worked wonders for you; never again will my people be shamed.

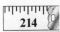

214

Joel 2:12-13 (NASB)

¹² "Yet even now," declares the Lord, "Return to Me with all your heart, And with fasting, weeping and mourning; ¹³ And rend your heart and not your garments."
Now return to the Lord your God, For He is gracious and compassionate, Slow to anger, abounding in loving kindness and relenting of evil.

1 Corinthians 3:17b (NLT)

...For God's temple is holy, and you are that temple.

John 8:34 (NIV)

³⁴ Jesus replied, "Very truly I tell you, everyone who sins is a slave to sin."

Hebrews 3:15 (NIV)

¹⁵ As has just been said:
"Today, if you hear his voice, do not harden your hearts as you did in the rebellion."

1 Corinthians 6:19-20 (NIV)

¹⁹ Do you not know that your bodies are temples of the Holy Spirit, who is in you, whom you have received from God? You are not your own; ²⁰ you were bought at a price. Therefore honor God with your bodies.

Exodus 15:22-24 (NIV)

²² Then Moses led Israel from the Red Sea and they went into the Desert of Shur. For three days they traveled in the desert without finding water. ²³ When they came to Marah, they could not drink its water because it was bitter. (That is why the place is called Marah.) ²⁴ So the people grumbled against Moses, saying, "What are we to drink?"

Matthew 4:4 (NIV)

⁴ Jesus answered, "It is written: 'Man shall not live on bread alone, but on every word that comes from the mouth of God.'"

Psalm 119:103 (NIV)

¹⁰³ How sweet are your words to my taste, sweeter than honey to my mouth!

Psalm 119:2 (NIV)

² Blessed are those who keep his statutes and seek him with all their heart—

Psalm 119:105 (MSG)

¹⁰⁵⁻¹¹² By your words I can see where I'm going; they throw a beam of light on my dark path.

Psalm 119:25 (NIV)

²⁵ I am laid low in the dust; preserve my life according to your word.

Proverbs 23:20-21 (NIV)

²⁰ Do not join those who drink too much wine or gorge themselves on meat, ²¹ for drunkards and gluttons become poor, and drowsiness clothes them in rags.

2 Timothy 1:7 (NIV)

⁷ For the Spirit God gave us does not make us timid, but gives us power, love and self-discipline.

1 Corinthians 10:13 (MSG)

¹³ No test or temptation that comes your way is beyond the course of what others have had to face. All you need to remember is that God will never let you down; he'll never let you be pushed past your limit; he'll always be there to help you come through it.

Psalm 81:8-10 (NIV)   *⁸ Hear me, my people, and I will warn you— if you would only listen to me, Israel!*
⁹ You shall have no foreign god among you; you shall not worship any god other than me.
¹⁰ I am the Lord your God, who brought you up out of Egypt.
Open wide your mouth and I will fill it.

James 1:14-15 (NIV)   *¹⁴ but each person is tempted when they are dragged away by their own evil desire and enticed. ¹⁵ Then, after desire has conceived, it gives birth to sin...*

Proverbs 14:16 (NASB)   *¹⁶ A wise man...turns away from evil, But a fool is arrogant and careless.*

Psalm 119:59-60 (NIV)   *⁵⁹ I have considered my ways and have turned my steps to your statutes. ⁶⁰ I will hasten and not delay to obey your commands.*

Hebrews 4:15-16 (NIV)   *¹⁵ For we do not have a high priest who is unable to empathize with our weaknesses, but we have one who has been tempted in every way, just as we are—yet he did not sin. ¹⁶ Let us then approach God's throne of grace with confidence, so that we may receive mercy and find grace to help us in our time of need.*

Psalm 50:15a (NIV)   *¹⁵ and call on me in the day of trouble...*

James 5:16 (GW)	*16 So admit your sins to each other...so that you will be healed.*
Proverbs 14:16 (NASB)	*16 A wise man is cautious and turns away from evil, But a fool is arrogant and careless.*
Ephesians 4:27 (NIV)	*27 and do not give the devil a foothold.*
Ephesians 6:17 (NIV)	*17 Take the helmet of salvation and the sword of the Spirit, which is the word of God.*
Matthew 26:41a (NIV)	*41 "Watch and pray so that you will not fall into temptation.*
1 Corinthians 10:12 (NIV)	*12 So, if you think you are standing firm, be careful that you don't fall!*
Genesis 9:3 (NIV)	*3 Everything that lives and moves about will be food for you. Just as I gave you the green plants, I now give you everything.*
1 Timothy 4:1-5 (NASB)	*4 But the Spirit explicitly says that in later times some will fall away from the faith, paying attention to deceitful spirits and doctrines of demons, 2 by means of the hypocrisy of liars seared in their own conscience as with a branding iron, 3men who forbid marriage and advocate abstaining from foods which God has created to be gratefully shared in by those who believe and know the truth. 4 For everything created by God is good, and nothing is to be rejected if it is received with gratitude; 5 for it is sanctified by means of the word of God and prayer.*

218

Deuteronomy 12:15, 20, 21, 26 (NASB)

[15] *"However, you may slaughter and eat meat within any of your gates, whatever you desire, according to the blessing of the Lord your God which He has given you; the unclean and the clean may eat of it, as of the gazelle and the deer.* [20] *"When the Lord your God extends your border as He has promised you, and you say, 'I will eat meat,' because you desire to eat meat, then you may eat meat, whatever you desire.* [21] *If the place which the Lord your God chooses to put His name is too far from you, then you may slaughter of your herd and flock which the Lord has given you, as I have commanded you; and you may eat within your gates whatever you desire.* [26] *Only your holy things which you may have and your votive offerings, you shall take and go to the place which the Lord chooses.*

Mark 7:18-20 (NASB)

[18] *And He *said to them, "Are you so lacking in understanding also? Do you not understand that whatever goes into the man from outside cannot defile him,* [19] *because it does not go into his heart, but into his stomach, and is eliminated?" (Thus He declared all foods clean.)* [20] *And He was saying, "That which proceeds out of the man, that is what defiles the man.*

Genesis 1:29-30 (NIV)

[29] *Then God said, "I give you every seed-bearing plant on the face of the whole earth and every tree that has fruit with seed in it. They will be yours for food.* [30] *And to all the beasts of the earth and all the birds in the sky and all the creatures that move*

along the ground—everything that has the breath of life in it—I give every green plant for food." And it was so.

Acts 10:15 (NIV)   *"...Do not call anything impure that God has made clean."*

Romans 14:2-3, 6 (NIV)   *² One person's faith allows them to eat anything, but another, whose faith is weak, eats only vegetables. ³ The one who eats everything must not treat with contempt the one who does not, and the one who does not eat everything must not judge the one who does, for God has accepted them. ⁶ ...Whoever eats meat does so to the Lord, for they give thanks to God; and whoever abstains does so to the Lord and gives thanks to God.*

Proverbs 12:10a (NIV)   *¹⁰ The righteous care for the needs of their animals*

Isaiah 25:6 (NIV)   *⁶ On this mountain the Lord Almighty will prepare a feast of rich food for all peoples, a banquet of aged wine— the best of meats and the finest of wines.*

Genesis 1:30 (NRSV)   *³⁰ And to every beast of the earth, and to every bird of the air, and to everything that creeps on the earth, everything that has the breath of life, I have given every green plant for food." And it was so.*

Daniel 1:8, 11-12, 15 (NIV)

But Daniel resolved not to defile himself with the royal food and wine...
Daniel then said..."Give us nothing but vegetables to eat and water to drink...At the end of the ten days they looked healthier and better nourished than any of the young men who ate the royal food.

Isaiah 65:25 (NRSV)

25 The wolf and the lamb shall feed together, the lion shall eat straw like the ox; but the serpent—its food shall be dust!
They shall not hurt or destroy on all my holy mountain, says the LORD.

Job 12:7 (NRSV)

7 "But ask the animals, and they will teach you; the birds of the air, and they will tell you;

Proverbs 12:10 (NRSV)

10 The righteous know the needs of their animals, but the mercy of the wicked is cruel.

Psalm 147:9 (NRSV)

9 He gives to the animals their food, and to the young ravens when they cry.

Hosea 2:18 (NRSV)

18 I will make for you a covenant on that day with the wild animals, the birds of the air, and the creeping things of the ground; and I will abolish the bow, the sword, and war from the land; and I will make you lie down in safety.

Jeremiah 12:4 (NRSV)

4 How long will the land mourn, and the grass of every field wither?
For the wickedness of those who live in it the animals and the birds are swept away, and because people said, "He is blind to our ways."

221

Luke 12:6 (NRSV)   *⁶ Are not five sparrows sold for two pennies? Yet not one of them is forgotten in God's sight.*

Psalm 36:6 (NRSV)   *⁶ Your righteousness is like the mighty mountains, your judgments are like the great deep; you save humans and animals alike, O LORD.*

Matthew 5:7 (NRSV)   *⁷ "Blessed are the merciful, for they will receive mercy.*

1 Corinthians 10:23 (NIV)   *²³ "I have the right to do anything," you say—but not everything is beneficial. "I have the right to do anything"—but not everything is constructive.*

Matthew 11:18-19 (NIV)   *¹⁸ For John came neither eating nor drinking, and they say, 'He has a demon.' ¹⁹ The Son of Man came eating and drinking, and they say, 'Here is a glutton and a drunkard, a friend of tax collectors and sinners.' But wisdom is proved right by her deeds."*

2 Corinthians 10:5-6 (NIV)   *⁵ We demolish arguments and every pretension that sets itself up against the knowledge of God, and we take captive every thought to make it obedient to Christ. 6 And we will be ready to punish every act of disobedience, once your obedience is complete.*

Matthew 9:15 (NIV)   *¹⁵ Jesus answered, "How can the guests of the bridegroom mourn while he is with them? The time will come when the bridegroom will be taken from them; then they will fast.*

Acts 13:2 (NIV)

2 While they were worshiping the Lord and fasting, the Holy Spirit said, "Set apart for me Barnabas and Saul for the work to which I have called them."

Acts 14:23 (NIV)

23 Paul and Barnabas appointed elders for them in each church and, with prayer and fasting, committed them to the Lord, in whom they had put their trust.

Philippians 4:8 (NIV)

8 Finally, brothers and sisters, whatever is true, whatever is noble, whatever is right, whatever is pure, whatever is lovely, whatever is admirable—if anything is excellent or praiseworthy—think about such things.

Proverbs 12:5 (NIV)

5 The plans of the righteous are just, but the advice of the wicked is deceitful.

John 15:5 (NIV)

5 "I am the vine; you are the branches. If you remain in me and I in you, you will bear much fruit; apart from me you can do nothing.

Galatians 4:9 (NIV)

9 But now that you know God—or rather are known by God—how is it that you are turning back to those weak and miserable forces? Do you wish to be enslaved by them all over again?

James 4:7 (NIV)

7 Submit yourselves, then, to God. Resist the devil, and he will flee from you.

Proverbs 29:18 (NIV)

18 Where there is no revelation, people cast off restraint; but blessed is the one who heeds wisdom's instruction.

1 Timothy 4:8 (NIV)　　　*⁸ For physical training is of some value*

Proverbs 23:7 (NKJV)　　*⁷ For as he thinks in his heart, so is he... Whatever you think of yourself is how you will turn out.*

Proverbs 4:23 (NCV)　　*²³ Be careful what you think, because your thoughts run your life.*

Job 3:25 (MSG)　　*²⁵ The worst of my fears has come true, what I've dreaded most has happened.*

Daniel 9:3-5 (NASB)　　*³So I gave my attention to the Lord God to seek Him by prayer and supplications, with fasting, sackcloth and ashes. 4 I prayed to the Lord my God and confessed and said, "Alas, O Lord, the great and awesome God, who keeps His covenant and lovingkindness for those who love Him and keep His commandments, 5 we have sinned, committed iniquity, acted wickedly and rebelled, even turning aside from Your commandments and ordinances.*

1 Corinthians 9:27 (NLT)　　*²⁷ I discipline my body like an athlete, training it to do what it should.*

Philippians 3:19-20 (NLT)　　*¹⁹ They are headed for destruction. Their god is their appetite, they brag about shameful things, and they think only about this life here on earth. ²⁰ But we are citizens of heaven, where the Lord Jesus Christ lives. And we are eagerly waiting for him to return as our Savior.*

Proverbs 25:28 (NIV)　　*²⁸ Like a city whose walls are broken through is a person who lacks self-control.*

Scripture References

Psalm 81:16 (NLT)

16 But I would feed you with the finest wheat. I would satisfy you with wild honey from the rock."

Exodus 16:1-5 (NIV)

The whole Israelite community set out from Elim and came to the Desert of Sin, which is between Elim and Sinai, on the fifteenth day of the second month after they had come out of Egypt. 2 In the desert the whole community grumbled against Moses and Aaron. 3 The Israelites said to them, "If only we had died by the Lord's hand in Egypt! There we sat around pots of meat and ate all the food we wanted, but you have brought us out into this desert to starve this entire assembly to death." 4 Then the Lord said to Moses, "I will rain down bread from heaven for you. The people are to go out each day and gather enough for that day. In this way I will test them and see whether they will follow my instructions. 5 On the sixth day they are to prepare what they bring in, and that is to be twice as much as they gather on the other days."

Acts 10:9-16 (NIV)

9 About noon the following day as they were on their journey and approaching the city, Peter went up on the roof to pray. 10 He became hungry and wanted something to eat, and while the meal was being prepared, he fell into a trance. 11 He saw heaven opened and something like a large sheet being let down to earth by its four corners. 12 It contained all kinds of four-footed animals, as well as reptiles and birds. 13 Then a voice told him, "Get up, Peter. Kill and eat."

14 "Surely not, Lord!" Peter replied. "I have never eaten anything impure or unclean."

15 The voice spoke to him a second time, "Do not call anything impure that God has made clean." 16 This happened three times, and immediately the sheet was taken back to heaven.

Leviticus 11: 1-8 (NIV)

11 The LORD said to Moses and Aaron, 2 "Say to the Israelites: 'Of all the animals that live on land, these are the ones you may eat: 3 You may eat any animal that has a divided hoof and that chews the cud.

4 There are some that only chew the cud or only have a divided hoof, but you must not eat them. The camel, though it chews the cud, does not have a divided hoof; it is ceremonially unclean for you. 5 The hyrax, though it chews the cud, does not have a divided hoof; it is unclean for you. 6 The rabbit, though it chews the cud, does not have a divided hoof; it is unclean for you. 7 And the pig, though it has a divided hoof, does not chew the cud; it is unclean for you. 8 You must not eat their meat or touch their carcasses; they are unclean for you.

Romans 14:14 (NIV)

14 I am convinced, being fully persuaded in the Lord Jesus, that nothing is unclean in itself. But if anyone regards something as unclean, then for that person it is unclean.

1 Corinthians 3:16 (NIV)

16 Don't you know that you yourselves are God's temple and that God's Spirit dwells in your midst?

Ephesians 5:18 (NIV)

18 Do not get drunk on wine, which leads to debauchery. Instead, be filled with the Spirit,

Proverbs 27:7 (NIV)

*7 One who is full loathes honey from the comb,
but to the hungry even what is bitter tastes sweet.*

**1 Corinthians 6:12b
(NIV)**

*12 "I have the right to do anything"—but I will not
be mastered by anything.*

Numbers 9:15-23 (NIV)

*15 On the day the tabernacle, the tent of the covenant
law, was set up, the cloud covered it. From evening
till morning the cloud above the tabernacle looked
like fire. 16 That is how it continued to be; the
cloud covered it, and at night it looked like fire.
17 Whenever the cloud lifted from above the tent,
the Israelites set out; wherever the cloud settled,
the Israelites encamped. 18 At the Lord's command
the Israelites set out, and at his command they
encamped. As long as the cloud stayed over the
tabernacle, they remained in camp. 19 When the
cloud remained over the tabernacle a long time,
the Israelites obeyed the Lord's order and did
not set out. 20 Sometimes the cloud was over the
tabernacle only a few days; at the Lord's command
they would encamp, and then at his command they
would set out. 21 Sometimes the cloud stayed only
from evening till morning, and when it lifted in the
morning, they set out. Whether by day or by night,
whenever the cloud lifted, they set out. 22 Whether
the cloud stayed over the tabernacle for two days
or a month or a year, the Israelites would remain in
camp and not set out; but when it lifted, they would
set out. 23 At the Lord's command they encamped,
and at the Lord's command they set out. They
obeyed the Lord's order, in accordance with his
command through Moses.*

Withdrawn

CPSIA information can be obtained
at www.ICGtesting.com
Printed in the USA
LVHW05s0533140418
573475LV00013BB/671/P